I0711944

ISBN: 9798746790897

60-DAY
SENIOR MEN
1200-CALORIE

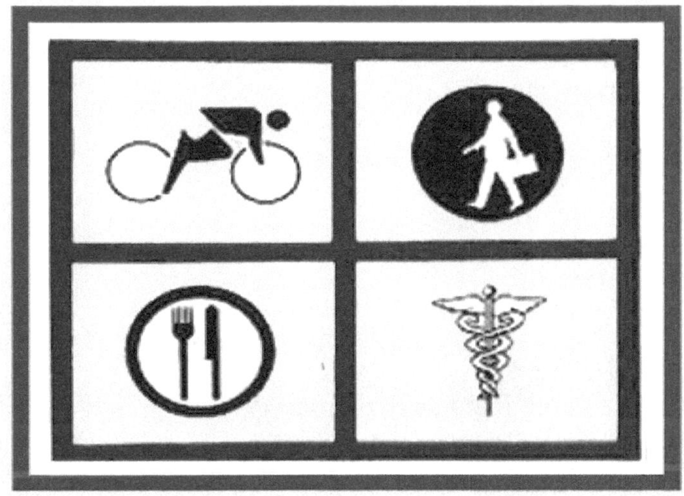

Vincent Antonetti, PhD

NoPaperPress™

NOTE: At publication, the off-the-shelf foods used in portions of this book were widely available in most supermarkets. But food products come and go. So if there is a frozen entrée or soup selection in this diet that is out of stock, or that's been discontinued, or perhaps that you don't like, or that you forgot to pick up while shopping, please substitute another food that has **approximately** the same caloric value and nutritional content. In this regard, many dieters have found the foods listed in the Appendices at the end of this book to be very helpful.

CONTENTS

Day 18 – Grilled Swordfish (94)
Day 19 – Chinese Dinner Out (95)
Day 20 – Quick Pasta Puttanesca (96)
Day 21 – Frozen Meat Dinner (97)
Day 22 – Shrimp & Spinach Salad (98)
Day 23 – Beans & Greens Salad (99)
Day 24 – Four Beans Plus Salad (100)
Day 25 – Pan-Broiled Hanger Steak (101)
Day 26 – Grilled Scallops & Polenta (102)
Day 27 – Fettuccine in Summer Sauce (103)
Day 28 – Frozen Chicken Dinner (104)
Day 29 – Barbequed Shrimp & Corn (105)
Day 30 – Cheeseburger Heaven (106)
Day 31 – Baked Sea Bass (107)
Day 32 – Grilled Turkey Tenders (108)
Day 33 – Frozen Fish Dinner (109)
Day 34 – Pasta Rapini (110)
Day 35 – Chicken Dinner Out (111)
Day 36 – Grilled Tilapia (112)
Day 37 – Lo-Cal Beef Stew (113)
Day 38 – Broiled Lamb Chop (114)
Day 39 – Chicken with Veggies (115)
Day 40 – Fish Dinner Out (116)
Day 41 – Pasta e Fagioli (117)
Day 42 – Muffins (118)
Day 43 – Beef Kebob (119)
Day 44 – Baked Haddock (120)
Day 45 – Chicken Cacciatore (121)
Day 46 – Poached Cod (122
Day 47 – Chinese Dinner Out (123)
Day 48 – Healthy Pasta Salad (124)
Day 49 – Frozen Meat Dinner (125)
Day 50 – Pan-Fried Sole (126)
Day 51 – Beans & Greens Salad (127)
Day 52 – Chicken Piccata (128)
Day 53 – Beef Steak Strips (129)
Day 54 – Grilled Scallops & Polenta (130)
Day 55 – Hearty Vegetable Soup (131)
Day 56 – Frozen Chicken Dinner (132)
Day 57 – Salmon with Mango Salsa (133)

The Best Weight Loss Diets

According to the late Dr. Jean Mayer, of Tufts University's Department of Nutrition, a really good weight-loss diet must have the following three characteristics:

1) The diet must provide you with an understanding of weight control as well as the knowledge you need to reduce your weight to the desired level.

2) The diet must help you remain healthy while you are losing weight.

3) The diet must lead you to a healthier way of eating and exercising that

Why You Lose Weight

Most experts agree that when the energy value of the food you eat minus waste, equals the sum of your basal metabolic energy plus the energy you expend during physical activity, you will neither gain nor lose weight. They also agree that when you have an energy imbalance, you will either gain or lose weight. In general then:

- **Weight Maintenance** occurs when your food energy intake equals the total energy you expend in daily living. In this case your weight remains stable, i.e., you neither gain nor lose weight.

- **Weight Gain** occurs when your food energy intake is greater than the total energy you expend in daily living. In this case your body stores the extra energy as fat.

- **Weight Loss** occurs when your food energy intake is less than the total energy you expend in daily living. In this case your body converts stored fat (and in some cases muscle) into energy.

The measure of energy, whether in the form of food, physical activity, or heat, is the kilocalorie (hereafter simply called the Calorie). As already mentioned, weight loss occurs when you eat fewer calories than the calories you use in your day-to-day living. This difference in calories is referred to as your calorie deficit. How much weight you lose depends on the magnitude of your calorie deficit. (In technical terms, **the calorie deficit, or calorie difference, is the driving force for weight change**.)

Most people on a weight-loss diet want to know how much weight they will lose – and how fast. Simple metabolic calculations make a rough estimate possible. Physiologists have long known that to lose one pound requires a deficit of approximately 3500 Calories. Therefore, if a person's total calorie deficit over time is known, their weight loss over time can be calculated. (See "**Expected Weight Loss**" - page 8.) **In summary, if you eat and exercise such that you have a calorie deficit you will lose weight!**

Expected Weight Loss

On the *60-Day Diet - 1200 Calorie Edition*, <u>**most senior men lose 27 to 36 pounds.**</u> Smaller men, older men (over 65) and less active men lose a bit less and larger men, younger men and more active men often lose more.

Exactly how much weight you will lose depends on how much you weigh, your age and your activity level. For the full story see *Weight Control - U.S. Edition* by Vincent W. Antonetti, Ph.D., an eBook also published by NoPaperPress.

First a Medical Exam

Everyone should at the very least have a medical assessment, or exam, before starting a weight loss diet. Why? You need to make sure your health will allow you to lower your caloric intake and increase your physical activity. Depending on your age and state of health, the medical checkup may be as simple as a visit to a physician who is familiar with your medical history, or it may be a thorough physical exam. The physician conducting the medical exam should be made aware of and should approve the specific weight loss diet you're planning. Additionally, if you are going to engage in some sort of physical activity in conjunction with this diet and especially if you have been totally inactive, or if you have or suspect you have cardiovascular disease or other health problems, or if you are obese, or if you are 40 or older, before embarking on the physical fitness portion of your weight control program you should have a stress test supervised by a physician. Finally, your physician can tell you how much and what type of exercise is right for you, how much you
should weigh, and prescribe a realistic weight- loss goal.

Eat Smart

No single food can supply all the nutrients you need in the amounts you need. The most important factors in nutrition are variety, variety, variety! **Variety is the key to a nutritious diet.** As a means of setting strategies for food selection, the U.S. Department of Health and Human Services and the Department of Agriculture issue

Dietary Guidelines every five years. The latest Dietary Guidelines describe a healthy diet as one that:
- Emphasizes fruits, vegetables, whole grains, and fat-free or low-fat milk products.
- Includes fish, poultry, lean meats, beans and nuts.
- Is low in saturated fats, trans fats, cholesterol, salt (sodium) and added sugars.
The latest guidelines encourage adults to consume a variety of nutrient-dense foods and beverages within their caloric needs. The afore mentioned U.S. government agencies recommend how much should be eaten from each of the basic food groups (i.e., from the fruit group, vegetable group, grains group, meat and beans group, dairy group, and oils group) to meet your caloric goal – whether you are trying to lose weight or maintain weight. All this information and more can be found in *Eat Smart - U.S. Edition* an eBook published by NoPaperPress.

Even though most adults can get all the vitamins and minerals they need by merely consuming a variety of nutritious foods (from the fruit group, the vegetable group, the grains group, the meat and beans group, the milk group, and the oils group), many physicians recommend a daily multi-vitamin/mineral supplement – just in case you don't eat the way you should.

Be aware that some micronutrients, such as the fat-soluble vitamin A, can be harmful if taken in large quantities. To be safe your multi-vitamin/mineral supplement should contain no more than 100 percent of the recommended dietary allowance (RDA) for each vitamin or mineral. Generally, you don't need the high doses in multi-vitamin/mineral supplements labeled "therapeutic" or "extra-strength." There may be medical reasons for taking larger amounts of a vitamin or mineral than the RDA provides, but check with your doctor first.

Tossed Salad

One of the dinner mainstays in the *60-Day Diet* is a "Tossed Salad." To prepare your "Tossed Salad" start with a bowl that has a volume of <u>at least</u> 16 ounces, or 2 cups. First add about 1 cup of either green leaf lettuce, Romaine lettuce or a Mesclun mix. Then add at least a half cup of other veggies such as broccoli, celery, cucumber, spinach, or watercress. This combination will total about 35 Calories

You'll be eating a "Tossed Salad" just about every day at dinnertime. Remember that variety is the key to a nutritious diet. So be sure to vary the ingredients of the salad. Top your Tossed Salad with 1½ tablespoons of any light salad dressing available at your local supermarket that contains no more than 25 Calories per tablespoon. Some of our favorites are:
- **Ken's Steakhouse Fat Free Raspberry Pecan**
- **Kraft Light Done Right House Italian**
- **Newman's Lighten Up! Balsamic Vinaigrette**
- **Wishbone Just 2 Good Honey Dijon**
Your "Tossed Salad" with salad dressing will cost you roughly 70 Calories but will be packed with lots of health-giving vitamins, minerals and fiber.

Regarding Bread

First understand that bread, more specifically whole-grain breads, are good sources of complex carbohydrates and dietary fiber, as well as the B vitamins (thiamin, riboflavin, niacin, and folate), vitamin E, and minerals (iron, magnesium and selenium). In recent years, however, sliced bread loaves have gotten larger, as have the bread slices inside these loaves. Just a few years ago the standard slice of bread contained about 65 to 70 Calories – now most are 100 plus Calories.

The 60-*Day Diet* requires whole-grain bread at 70 Calories per slice. Quite a few bakers sell thin sliced or "light" sliced bread. The difficult part is finding a whole grain thin sliced or "light" bread (with about 70 Calories per slice). Whatever the brand, make sure the first word in the Ingredients list is "whole." "Pepperidge Farm Small Slice 100% Whole Wheat" is a good choice. It's whole grain, has 70 Calories per slice and it tastes good too.

Substituting Foods

If there is a food listed in the *60-Day Diet* that you don't like, or perhaps that you forgot to pick up while shopping, you probably can exchange or substitute another food in its place – a technique used by dieticians. Exchanging a food listed in a diet for another food with approximately equal caloric value and nutritional content is the foundation of many successful long-term diets. Substitution possibilities are almost endless but have to be done carefully. The easiest substitutions are those within the same food group, such as exchanging one vegetable variety for another, or a glass of milk for a cup of yogurt. More sophisticated exchanges cross food groups, such as replacing 3½ ounces of turkey with a tablespoon of peanut butter on a piece of whole-wheat bread. Both foods are complete protein and both contain about 175 Calories. (Refer to a good online calorie table.) With some understanding and experience, you can use a calorie table to help you substitute foods called for in the *60-Day Diet* with equal calorie foods from the same food group.

Breakfast: You may substitute any cereal for any other wholesome cereal. For example, if you're not crazy about having Shredded Wheat for breakfast on Day 6, substitute Wheat Chex or Cheerios, etc. But remember to adjust the amount of cereal to account for the calorie difference between brands. If you don't like the soft-boiled egg called for on Day 9, cook a fried egg instead. And if Cantaloupe is on the menu but is not in season, replace cantaloupe with a half cup of orange juice – both contain about 50 Calories.

Snacks: Again, where 6 ounces of yogurt is specified you may substitute an 8-ounce glass of skim milk, but to maintain a nutritionally balanced diet keep this snack a dairy selection. Similarly, when fruit is on the agenda, you may select any type of fruit but do not stray from the fruit group. Nuts and popcorn can be interchanged at will. Specified convenient brand-name snacks, such as Skinny Cow ice cream, Kashi Granola bars, Nabisco 100 Calorie Pack cookies and Orville Redenbacher's Smart Pop Popcorn should be widely available but other equivalent brands may be substituted if need be. Just make sure the substitute snack has the same calorie count, or very close, to the specified snack.

Two Nights – No Cooking

Everyone deserves a break from the grind of preparing dinner after coming home from work. So the *60-Day Diet* gives you two days off per week! Notice that one night a week the meal plan calls for a frozen dinner and on a second night during the week you're encouraged to eat out. There are, however, some rules and caveats involved – these are covered in the next two sections.

Frozen Dinner Rules

In general, a frozen dinner should not be a meal in itself. Make sure you add a salad, fruit, bread etc. The frozen dinner you choose should come with at least one cup of cooked vegetables. If your frozen dinner doesn't measure up, add your own frozen, fresh or canned vegetables. And look for dinners with no more than 800 mg of sodium. In addition, make sure the dinner you choose has no more than 30 percent of the daily value for total fat. Appendix A on page 196 contains a comprehensive tabulation of reasonably good frozen dinner choices. And on the days when a frozen dinner is specified, you will be given a calorie goal for the frozen dinner. For example, Day 5 calls for frozen fish dinner with a maximum allowable 340 Calories. If you choose a frozen fish dinner that contains less than 340 Calories, you may spend the unused calories any way you wish.

Moreover, on those nights when you just don't have the energy or time to cook, you can always substitute a frozen dinner for the "Recipe of the Day" or the entree listed in the meal plan. For example, Day 2 calls for Herb-Crusted Cod for dinner. The total calorie count for dinner is 520. In place of the cod, any combination of a frozen fish dinner and side dishes (salads, etc) with a total calorie content close to 520 would be an acceptable, albeit not as tasty, alternative.

Eating Out Challenges

You may eat out once a week. When you're on a diet, however, eating in a restaurant can be a challenge, because most restaurant portions are huge, and can easily total more than 1000 Calories. On the *60-Day Diet*, a dinner type (i.e., fish, chicken, etc) and a calorie target is specified. For example Day 7 of the 1200 Calorie diet calls for a chicken dinner and allows you 530 Calories.

First, you need to choose a restaurant where you have a fighting chance to achieve your calorie goal. Next, order something simple, such as broiled fish with steamed vegetables and brown rice. Tell the waiter you want no sauce, no gravy, nothing added. Then, knowing your calorie objective, and that most fish and chicken are about 50 Calories per ounce, most steamed vegetable servings average approximately 50 Calories per cup, and rice is about 100 Calories per ½ cup, decide how much to eat and take the remainder home. If fresh fruit is not an option, pass on dessert and have the snack in the meal plan.

Important Notes

1) Coffee or tea may be caffeinated or decaf. If desired, skim milk and a sugar substitute may be added to coffee or tea, and **Soy or Almond** milk may be used instead of cow's milk.

2) Fried eggs or scrambled eggs should be cooked in a pan coated with a non-stick cooking spray. Hard-boiled eggs may be substituted for fried, scrambled or soft-boiled eggs.

3) Cereals should be whole grain and unsweetened. At the top of the list are Old-fashioned Oatmeal, Wheatena and Shredded Wheat. Among other reasonably healthy choices are Cheerios, Wheat Chex, Wheaties, some Kashi cereals and Farina. When blueberries are in season, you may **substitute blueberries for raisins** added to your cereal. (Approx. substitution ratio = 2 blueberries for one raisin.)

4) Bread may be either plain or toasted whole grain, such as whole wheat, whole rye or pumpernickel. Look for whole grain varieties that contain 70 Calories per slice. If desired, bread may be sprayed with a zero-calorie butter substitute.

5) When soup in a microwaveable bowl or a can is specified, eat only one serving (8 ounces) unless otherwise noted. (Microwaveable bowls and cans usually contain about two servings.)

6) Use freely as desired: clear unsweetened coffee, clear unsweetened tea, water, seltzer water and any diet soda, clear soups without fat, bouillon, and seasonings such as mustard, cinnamon, dill, herbs, red and black pepper, curry, vinegar, lemon juice and sections, and dill and sour pickles.

7) Use only lean cuts of meat trimmed of all visible fat. Poultry should be limited to chicken or turkey breasts (white meat only and skinless).

8) When canned tuna or salmon is specified, use fish **packed in water**.

9) When the diet calls for turkey bacon, make sure the brand you buy has no more than 35 Calories per slice.

10) An unlimited amount of green salad may be eaten, but the salad dressing should be as specified.

11) If it's more convenient, any food item may be moved to any part of the day and combined with any meal or snack.

12) If you cannot find the exact item called for in the diet (because it's out of stock or discontinued), substitute a comparable food (of the same type and close caloric value).

   13) Take a daily **multi-vitamin/mineral supplement**. This is important when you're on a diet – as a kind of insurance policy.

Keeping It Off

Within five years, more than 90 percent of all dieters regain every pound they have lost. Why? In most cases it's because after losing weight most people eventually revert to their pre-diet eating and exercising habits,
and this inevitably leads to their regaining the weight they lost – and often more. Obviously after a diet you weigh less. The fact is the less you weigh, the less you need to eat to sustain your lower weight.

A study, published in the *Annals of Internal Medicine*, that followed 4,000 people for three decades suggests that in the long term, 90 percent of men and 70 percent of women will become overweight. Interestingly, half of the men and women in the study, who had made it well into adulthood without a weight problem, ultimately also became overweight and a third actually became obese. The point being that you can never
become complacent. You must continually watch your weight because we are all at risk of becoming overweight.

The key to long-term weight control success is knowledge and understanding, combined of course with desire and self-discipline. Once you reach your weight goal, I suggest you read ***Weight Maintenance - U.S. Edition*** by Vincent Antonetti, Ph.D. (also published by NoPaperPress) – considered the best weight maintenance eBook, or paperback, on the market.

1200 CALORIE DAILY MENUS

Day 1 Daily Menu

BREAKFAST	Calories	Totals
Grapefruit (½)	75	
Scrambled egg (See Notes - page 13)	80	
Whole grain toast (1 slice) (page 13)	70	
Coffee (page 13)	10	235 Cal
SNACK		
Coffee or tea	10	10 Cal
LUNCH		
Ham (2 oz) with mustard on 2 slices rye bread	290	
Pickle spear	0	
Hot or iced tea	10	300 Cal
SNACK		
Fresh fruit in season (apple, peach, etc)	70	
Coffee or tea	10	80 Cal
DINNER		
Chicken with Peppers & Onions (**Recipe 1** page 77)	250	
Sautéed red peppers with onions (Recipe 1)	70	
Green beans (steamed) & mashed cauliflower	25	
Large tossed salad - 1½ Tbsp dressing (See page 10)	85	
Water with lemon wedge	15	475 Cal
SNACK		
Graham crackers (2 squares)	60	
Skim milk (4 oz = ½ cup)	45	105 Cal
		1205 Cal

Day 2 Daily Menu

BREAKFAST	Calories	Totals
Orange juice (½ cup)	50	
Wheaties (¾ cup) + ½ cup skim milk + ½ banana	190	
Coffee	10	250
SNACK		
Fresh fruit in season (apple, pear, etc)	70	
Coffee or tea	10	80 Cal
LUNCH		
Soup (Appendix B - page 137)	110	
Turkey breast (1 oz) on 1 slice rye bread (½ sandwich)	105	
Pickle spear	0	
Lettuce & tomato slices	20	
Hot or iced tea	10	245
SNACK		
Coffee or tea	10	10 Cal
DINNER		
Baked Herb-Crusted Cod (Recipe 2 - page 78)	230	
Spinach (½ cup) steamed with garlic & drizzled	100	
Asparagus (8 spears cooked & drained)	25	
Bakcd potato (medium size) (No Butter!)	100	
Whole grain bread (1 slice)	70	
Water	0	525
SNACK		
Fiber One Chocolate Fudge Brownie	90	
Coffee or tea	10	100
		1210

Day 3 Daily Menu

BREAKFAST	Calories	Totals
Fresh or frozen strawberries (½ cup)	25	
French toasted English Muffin Recipe 3 - page 79	270	
Light syrup (1 Tbsp)	30	
Coffee	10	335 Cal
SNACK		
Coffee or tea	10	10 Cal
LUNCH		
Salad (3 oz can tuna, 1 tsp Evoo, onions, celery)	175	
Rye bread (1 slice)	70	
Small bunch of grapes	65	
Coffee or tea	10	320 Cal
SNACK		
Coffee or tea	10	10 Cal
DINNER		
Broiled veal chop (4 oz lean)	200	
Corn on the cob (1 medium ear) (No Butter!)	100	
Broccoli (½ cup steamed & drizzled with 1 tsp	70	
Large tossed salad - 1½ Tbsp dressing (See page 10)	85	
Fresh fruit in season (apple, peach, etc)	70	
Water	0	525 Cal
SNACK		
Coffee or tea	10	10 Cal
		1210 Cal

Day 4 Daily Menu

BREAKFAST	Calories	Totals
Grapefruit (½)	75	
Cheerios (1 cup) + ½ cup skim milk + about 15	190	
Coffee	10	275 Cal
SNACK		
Coffee or tea	10	10 Cal
LUNCH		
Cottage cheese (1 cup low fat)	180	
Large tossed salad with 1½ Tbsp low-cal	70	
Small whole-grain roll	80	
Water	0	330 Cal
SNACK		
Fresh fruit in season (peach, plum, etc)	70	
Coffee or tea	10	80 Cal
DINNER		
Meat Loaf (Recipe 4 - page 80)	290	
One-half acorn squash (baked with ½ tsp maple	60	
Spinach (½ cup steamed & drizzled with 1 tsp Evoo)	85	
Romaine lettuce, tomato slices, & 1 Tbsp low-cal	45	
Water	0	495 Cal
SNACK		
Coffee or tea	10	10 Cal
* See Notes - page 13 re substituting blueberries for		1200 Cal

Day 5 Daily Menu

BREAKFAST	Calories	Totals
Cantaloupe (½ medium)	50	
Fried egg	80	
Toasted raisin bread (1 slice)	75	
Coffee	10	215 Cal
SNACK		
Coffee or tea	10	10 Cal
LUNCH		
Subway 6" (Roast Beef, Cheese + veggies)*	245	
Large tossed salad with 1½ Tbsp low-cal	70	
Hot or iced tea	10	325 Cal
* On 6" half wheat roll.		
SNACK		
Yogurt (6 oz nonfat, any flavor)*	90	
Coffee or tea	10	100 Cal
DINNER		
Frozen fish dinner (Recipe 5 - page 81)	340	
Large tossed salad with 1½ Tbsp low-cal	70	
Whole-grain bread (1 slice)	70	
Fresh fruit in season (apple, peach, etc)	70	
Water	0	550 Cal
SNACK		
Coffee or tea	10	10 Cal
* For example, Dannon Lite & Fit. Buy 32 oz use 6 oz.		1210 Cal

Day 6 Daily Menu

BREAKFAST	Calories	Totals
Tomato juice (½ cup)	20	
Shredded Wheat (1 cup) + ½ cup milk + ½ banana	265	
Coffee	10	295 Cal
SNACK		
Coffee or tea	10	10 Cal
LUNCH		
Leftover meat loaf (½ of Recipe 4) with ketchup	155	
Small whole-grain roll	80	
Lettuce	0	
Fresh or frozen berries (½ cup)	50	
Water	0	285 Cal
SNACK		
Coffee or tea	10	10 Cal
DINNER		
Pizza (Recipe 6 - page 82)	350	
Large tossed salad with 1½ Tbsp low-cal	85	
Fresh fruit in season (apple, plum, etc)	70	
Water	0	550 Cal
SNACK		
Yogurt (4 oz, non-fat any flavor)*	60	
Coffee or tea	10	70 Cal
* Such as Dannon Lite & Fit. Buy 32 oz container use 6 oz.		1210 Cal

<u>Day 7 Daily Menu</u>

BREAKFAST	Calories	Totals
Cantaloupe (½ medium)	50	
Oatmeal ½ cup dry + ½ cup skim milk + about 15	220	
Coffee	10	280 Cal
SNACK		
Coffee or tea	10	10 Cal
LUNCH		
Soup (Appendix B - page 137)	90	
Grilled cheese sandwich (2 slices 2% cheese)	240	
Lettuce and sliced tomato	20	
Pickle spear	0	
Hot or iced tea	10	360 Cal
SNACK		
Coffee or tea	10	10 Cal
DINNER		
Eat Out – Chicken dinner (Recipe 7 - page 83)		
Max allowable calories	530	
Water	0	530 Cal
SNACK		
Coffee or tea	10	10 Cal
		1200 Cal

Day 8 Daily Menu

BREAKFAST	Calories	Totals
Cantaloupe (½ medium)	50	
Wheaties (¾ cup) + ½ cup skim milk + ½ banana	190	
Coffee	10	250 Cal
SNACK		
Fresh fruit in season (peach, plum, etc)	70	
Coffee or tea	10	80 Cal
LUNCH		
Soup (Appendix B - page 137)	130	
Turkey (1 oz) on 1 slice rye bread (½ sandwich)	120	
Lettuce & tomato slices	20	
Hot or iced tea	10	280 Cal
SNACK		
Coffee or tea	10	10 Cal
DINNER		
Baked salmon with salsa (Recipe 8 - page 84)	215	
Baked summer squash and zucchini	40	
Medium tomato - sliced	20	
Brown rice (½ cup – after cooking)	100	
Large tossed salad with 1½ Tbsp low-cal	70	
Water with lemon wedge	10	455 Cal
SNACK		
Graham crackers (3 squares)	90	
Skim milk (4 oz)	45	135 Cal
		1210 Cal

Day 9 Daily Menu

BREAKFAST	Calories	Totals
Orange juice (½ cup)	50	
Soft-boiled egg	80	
Whole grain toast (1 slice)	70	
Coffee	10	210 Cal
SNACK		
Yogurt (6 oz nonfat, any flavor)	90	
Coffee or tea	10	100 Cal
LUNCH		
Salad (3 oz canned tuna, 1 tsp Evoo, onions, celery)	175	
Lettuce & tomato wedges + rye bread (1 slice)	90	
Coffee or tea	10	275 Cal
SNACK		
Handful unsalted mixed nuts	100	
Coffee or tea	10	110 Cal
DINNER		
Veggie burger – (1 patty) (Recipe 9 - page 85)	100	
Low-fat cheddar cheese (1 thin slice)	50	
Seeded hamburger roll	140	
Beets (3 small, boiled, skinned & sliced)	45	
Fresh fruit in season (apple, peach, etc)	70	
Water	0	405 Cal
SNACK		
100-Calorie Pack Cookies	100	
Coffee or tea	10	110 Cal
		1210 Cal

Day 10 Daily Menu

BREAKFAST	Calories	Totals
Orange juice (½ cup)	50	
Wild blueberry pancakes (Recipe 10 - page 86)	190	
Light syrup (1½ Tbsp)	45	
Coffee	10	295 Cal
SNACK		
Coffee or tea	10	10 Cal
LUNCH		
Peanut butter 2 Tbsp on 2 slices whole-grain bread	340	
Skim milk (6 oz)	65	
Fresh fruit in season (apple, plum, etc)	70	475 Cal
SNACK		
Coffee or tea	10	10 Cal
DINNER		
Broiled pork chop about 4 oz of meat - trimmed of	260	
Green peas (½ cup)	55	
Tomato & cucumber salad with 1½ Tbsp low-cal	70	
Water with lemon wedge	10	395 Cal
SNACK		
Coffee or tea	10	10 Cal
		1195 Cal

Day 11 Daily Menu

BREAKFAST	Calories	Totals
Fresh sliced orange	75	
Cheerios (1 cup) + ½ cup skim milk + 15 raisins	190	
Coffee	10	275 Cal
SNACK		
Coffee or tea	10	10 Cal
LUNCH		
Ham & Cheddar*	270	
Fresh fruit in season (apple, plum, etc)	70	
Diet soda or water	0	340 Cal
* Hot Pockets (wrap) or an equivalent food.		
SNACK		
Handful unsalted mixed nuts	100	
Coffee or tea	10	110 Cal
DINNER		
Grilled chicken sausage (2 links 2½ oz per link)	180	
Artichoke-bean salad (Recipe 11 - page 87)	190	
Green beans (¼ lb – steamed)	25	
Whole-grain bread (1 slice)	70	
Water	0	465 Cal
SNACK		
Coffee or tea	10	10 Cal
		1210 Cal

Day 12   Daily Menu

BREAKFAST	Calories	Totals
Orange juice (½ cup)	50	
Scrambled egg	80	
Whole-grain toast (1 slice)	70	
Coffee	10	210 Cal
SNACK		
Yogurt (6 oz nonfat, any flavor)	90	
Coffee or tea	10	100 Cal
LUNCH		
Soup (Appendix B - page 137)	150	
Tomato slices w ¼ cup chopped basil + 1 tsp Evoo	60	
Whole-grain bread (1 slice)	70	
Hot or iced tea	10	290 Cal
SNACK		
Coffee or tea	10	10 Cal
DINNER		
Eat Out – Fish dinner (Recipe 12 - page 88)		
Max allowable calories	595	595 Cal
SNACK		
Coffee or tea	10	10 Cal
		1215 Cal

Day 13 Daily Menu

BREAKFAST	Calories	Totals
Orange juice (½ cup)	50	
Shredded Wheat (1 cup) + ½ cup + ½ banana	260	
Coffee	10	320 Cal
## SNACK		
Handful unsalted mixed nuts	100	
Coffee or tea	10	110 Cal
## LUNCH		
Turkey frank (2 oz) with mustard & relish	150	
Hot-dog bun	130	
Hot or iced tea	10	290 Cal
## SNACK		
Coffee or tea	10	10 Cal
## DINNER		
Pasta w Marinara sauce (**Recipe 13** - page 89)	225	
Large tossed salad w 1½ Tbsp low-cal dressing	70	
Fresh fruit in season (peach, plum, etc)	70	
Italian or French bread (1 slice)	80	
Water with lemon wedge	10	455 Cal
## SNACK		
Coffee or tea	10	10 Cal
		1195 Cal

Day 14 Daily Menu

BREAKFAST	Calories	Totals
Cantaloupe (½ medium)	50	
Low-Cal Smoothie (Recipe 14 - page 90)	220	
Coffee	10	280 Cal
SNACK		
Fresh fruit in season (apple, peach, etc)	70	
Coffee or tea	10	80 Cal
LUNCH		
Grilled Swiss cheese sandwich (2 oz low-fat cheese)	320	
Pickle spear	0	
Hot or iced tea	10	330 Cal
SNACK		
Coffee or tea	10	10 Cal
DINNER		
Frozen chicken dinner (Day 28 Recipe - page 104)	300	
Large tossed salad w 1½ Tbsp low-cal dressing	70	
Water with lemon wedge	10	380 Cal
SNACK		
Popcorn Mini Bag*	110	
Coffee or tea	10	120 Cal
* Such as Orville Redenbacher's Smart Pop		1200 Cal

Day 15 Daily Menu

BREAKFAST	Calories	Totals
Fresh or frozen strawberries (1 cup)	50	
French toasted English Muffin Recipe 3 - page 79	270	
Light syrup (1 Tbsp)	30	
Coffee	10	360 Cal
SNACK		
Yogurt (6 oz nonfat, any flavor)	90	
Coffee or tea	10	100 Cal
LUNCH		
Salad (3 oz canned tuna, 1 tsp Evoo, onions, celery)	175	
Rye bread (1 slice)	70	
Coffee or tea	10	255 Cal
SNACK		
Coffee or tea	10	10 Cal
DINNER		
London broil (Recipe 15 - page 91)	320	
Brown rice (½ cup – after cooking)	100	
Steamed broccoli (1 cup – after cooking)	50	
Water	0	470 Cal
SNACK		
Coffee or tea	10	10 Cal
		1205 Cal

Day 16 Daily Menu

BREAKFAST	Calories	Totals
Orange juice (½ cup)	50	
Kashi GoLean (1 cup) + ½ cup milk + ½ banana	235	
Coffee	10	295 Cal
SNACK		
Fresh fruit in season (apple, plum, etc)	70	
Coffee or tea	10	80 Cal
LUNCH		
Soup (Appendix B - page 137)	100	
Small whole-grain roll	80	
Lettuce and sliced tomato (with 1 Tbsp light mayo)	45	
Hot or iced tea	10	235 Cal
SNACK		
Coffee or tea	10	10 Cal
DINNER		
Baked red snapper (Recipe 16 - page 92)	215	
Wild rice mix (Recipe 16)	160	
Green beans & tomato	75	
Water	0	450 Cal
SNACK		
Popcorn Mini Bag	110	
Coffee or tea	10	120 Cal
		1190 Cal

Day 17 Daily Menu

BREAKFAST	Calories	Totals
Cantaloupe (½ medium)	50	
Fried egg	80	
Toasted raisin bread (1 slice)	75	
Coffee	10	215 Cal
SNACK		
Yogurt (6 oz nonfat, any flavor)	90	
Coffee or tea	10	100 Cal
LUNCH		
Hot Pockets Ham & Cheddar Wrap	270	
Fresh fruit in season (peach, plum, etc)	70	
Cucumber slices and carrots and celery sticks	15	
Hot or iced tea	10	365 Cal
SNACK		
Handful unsalted mixed nuts	100	
Coffee or tea	10	110 Cal
DINNER		
Cajun chicken salad (Recipe 17 - page 93)	330	
Whole-grain bread (1 slice)	70	
Water	0	400 Cal
SNACK		
Coffee or tea	10	10 Cal
		1200 Cal

<u>Day 18 Daily Menu</u>

BREAKFAST	Calories	Totals
Grapefruit (½)	**75**	
Cheerios (1 cup) + ½ cup skim milk + 15 raisins	**190**	
Coffee	**10**	**275 Cal**
<u>**SNACK**</u>		
Coffee or tea	**10**	**10 Cal**
<u>**LUNCH**</u>		
Subway 6" (Roast Beef, Cheese + veggies)*	**245**	
Water (or diet soda)	**0**	**245 Cal**
* On 6" half wheat roll.		
<u>**SNACK**</u>		
Handful unsalted mixed nuts	**100**	
Coffee or tea	**10**	**110 Cal**
<u>**DINNER**</u>		
Grilled swordfish (Recipe 18 - page 94)	**250**	
Grilled potatoes (Recipe 18)	**100**	
Grilled cherry tomatoes (Recipe 18)	**45**	
Spinach (½ cup) steamed w garlic & drizzled Evoo	**50**	
Water with lemon wedge	**10**	**455 Cal**
<u>**SNACK**</u>		
Fiber One Chocolate Fudge Brownie	**90**	
Coffee or tea	**10**	**100 Cal**
		1190 Cal

<u>Day 19 Daily Menu</u>

BREAKFAST	Calories	Totals
Grapefruit (½)	75	
Scrambled egg	80	
Whole-grain toast (1 slice)	70	
Coffee	10	235 Cal
SNACK		
Yogurt (6 oz nonfat, any flavor)	90	
Coffee or tea	10	100 Cal
LUNCH		
Soup (Appendix B - page 137)	90	
Turkey (1 oz) on 1 slice rye bread (½ sandwich)	120	210 Cal
Water	0	
SNACK		
Coffee or tea	10	10 Cal
DINNER		
Eat Out – Chinese food (Recipe 19 - page 95)*		
Max allowable calories	640	640 Cal
SNACK		
Coffee or tea	10	10 Cal
* Bring some home for Day 20 lunch.		1205 Cal

Day 20 Daily Menu

BREAKFAST	Calories	Totals
Tomato juice (½ cup)	20	
Shredded Wheat (1 cup) + ½ cup milk + ½ banana	260	
Coffee	10	290 Cal
SNACK		
Handful unsalted mixed nuts	100	
Coffee or tea	10	110 Cal
LUNCH		
Left over Chinese food from Day 19	260	
Hot or iced tea	10	270 Cal
SNACK		
Coffee or tea	10	10 Cal
DINNER		
Quick Pasta Puttanesca (Recipe 20 - page 96)	345	
Large tossed salad w 1½ Tbsp low-cal dressing	70	
Italian or French bread (1 slice)	80	
Water with lemon wedge	10	505 Cal
SNACK		
Coffee or tea	10	10 Cal
		1195 Cal

Day 21 Daily Menu

BREAKFAST	Calories	Totals
Cantaloupe (½ medium)	50	
Oatmeal ½ cup dry + ½ cup milk + about 15 raisins	220	
Coffee	10	280 Cal
SNACK		
Coffee or tea	10	10 Cal
LUNCH		
Turkey breast (2 oz) on 2 slices bread	245	
Lettuce, tomato and Tbsp light mayo	35	
Pickle spear	0	
Fresh fruit in season (peach, plum, etc)	70	
Water	0	350 Cal
SNACK		
Yogurt (6 oz nonfat, any flavor)	90	
Coffee or tea	10	100 Cal
DINNER		
Frozen meat dinner (Recipe 21 - page 97)	300	
Large tossed salad w 1½ Tbsp low-cal dressing	70	
Whole-grain bread (1 slice)	70	
Water with lemon wedge	10	450 Cal
SNACK		
Coffee or tea	10	10 Cal
		1200 Cal

Day 22 Daily Menu

BREAKFAST	Calories	Totals
Fresh or frozen strawberries (1 cup)	25	
French toasted English Muffin (Recipe 3 - page 109)	270	
Light syrup (1 Tbsp)	30	
Coffee	10	335 Cal
SNACK		
Coffee or tea	10	10 Cal
LUNCH		
Chorizo Egg & Cheese*	260	
Hot or iced tea	10	270 Cal
* Hot Pockets wrap or an equivalent food.		
SNACK		
Yogurt (6 oz nonfat, any flavor)	90	
Coffee or tea	10	100 Cal
DINNER		
Shrimp & spinach salad (Recipe 22 - page 98)	310	
Whole-grain bread (1 slice)	70	
Fresh fruit in season (apple, peach, etc)	70	
Water with lemon wedge	10	460 Cal
SNACK		
Coffee or tea	10	10 Cal
		1185 Cal

Day 23 Daily Menu

BREAKFAST	Calories	Totals
Cantaloupe (½ medium)	50	
Wheaties (¾ cup) + ½ cup skim milk + ½ banana	190	
Coffee	10	250 Cal
SNACK		
Handful unsalted mixed nuts	100	
Coffee or tea	10	110 Cal
LUNCH		
Ham (2 oz) w mustard on 2 slices rye bread	300	
Pickle spear	0	
Hot or iced tea	10	315 Cal
SNACK		
Coffee or tea	10	10 Cal
DINNER		
Beans & Greens Salad (Recipe 23 - page 99)	260	
Whole-grain bread (1 slice)	70	
Baked potato (medium)	100	
Fresh fruit in season (apple, plum, etc)	70	
Water	0	500 Cal
SNACK		
Coffee or tea	10	10 Cal
		1195 Cal

<h1 align="center"><u>Day 24 Daily Menu</u></h1>

BREAKFAST	Calories	Totals
Fresh orange sliced	75	
Soft-boiled egg	80	
Whole grain toast (1 slice)	70	
Coffee	10	235 Cal
SNACK		
Yogurt (6 oz nonfat, any flavor)	90	
Coffee or tea	10	100 Cal
LUNCH		
Salad 3 oz canned salmon, 1 tsp Evoo, onions celery	200	
Lettuce & tomato wedges	20	
Rye bread (1 slice)	70	
Coffee or tea	10	300 Cal
SNACK		
Fresh fruit in season (peach, plum, etc)	70	
Coffee or tea	10	80 Cal
DINNER		
Chicken breast (5 oz - skinless, broiled)	250	
Four bean salad (½ cup) (Recipe 24 - page 100)	135	
Large tossed salad with 1½ Tbsp low-cal	70	
Water with lemon wedge	10	465 Cal
SNACK		
Coffee or tea	10	10 Cal
		1190 Cal

Day 25 Daily Menu

BREAKFAST	Calories	Totals
Grapefruit (½)	75	
Cheerios (1 cup) + ½ cup skim milk + 15 raisins	190	
Coffee	10	275 Cal
SNACK		
Coffee or tea	10	10 Cal
LUNCH		
Cottage cheese (1 cup low fat)	180	
Large tossed salad w 1½ Tbsp low-cal dressing	70	
Small whole-grain roll	80	
Hot or iced tea	10	340 Cal
SNACK		
Coffee or tea	10	10 Cal
DINNER		
Hanger steak (Recipe 25 - page 101)	320	
Roasted potatoes (Recipe 25)	120	
Cherry tomatoes (Recipe 25)	20	
Steamed spinach (½ cup)	25	
Whole-grain bread (1 slice)	70	
Water	0	555 Cal
SNACK		
Coffee or tea	10	10 Cal
		1200 Cal

Day 26 Daily Menu

BREAKFAST	Calories	Totals
Cantaloupe (½ medium)	50	
Fried eggs (2 eggs)	160	
Toasted whole-grain bread (1 slice)	70	
Coffee	10	290 Cal
SNACK		
Yogurt (6 oz nonfat, any flavor)	90	
Coffee or tea	10	100 Cal
LUNCH		
Soup (Appendix B - page 137)	160	
Hard whole-grain roll (medium)	80	
Lettuce & tomato slices	20	
Hot or iced tea	10	270 Cal
SNACK		
Fresh fruit in season (apple, peach, etc)	70	
Coffee or tea	10	80 Cal
DINNER		
Grilled scallops (Recipe 26 - page 1002)	210	
Grilled polenta (Recipe 26)	125	
Mushroom-steamed green beans-red onion	45	
Grilled asparagus (all shown in Recipe 26)	10	
Large tossed salad w 1½ Tbsp low-cal dressing	70	
Water	0	460 Cal
SNACK		
Coffee or tea	10	10 Cal
		1210 Cal

Day 27 Daily Menu

BREAKFAST	Calories	Totals
Orange juice (½ cup)	50	
Oatmeal ½ cup dry + ½ cup skim milk + about 15	220	
Coffee	10	280 Cal
SNACK		
Coffee or tea	10	10 Cal
LUNCH		
Left over Bean Salad from Day 23 (1 serving)	260	
Small whole-grain roll	80	
Lettuce & tomato slices	20	
Hot or iced tea	10	370 Cal
SNACK		
Fresh fruit in season (apple, plum, etc)	70	
Coffee or tea	10	80 Cal
DINNER		
Fettuccine (Recipe 27 - page 103)	290	
Large tossed salad w 1½ Tbsp low-cal dressing	70	
Italian or French bread (1 slice)	80	
Water with lemon wedge	10	450 Cal
SNACK		
Coffee or tea	10	10 Cal
		1200 Cal

Day 28 Daily Menu

BREAKFAST	Calories	Totals
Cantaloupe (½ medium)	50	
Smoothie (Recipe 14 - page 90)	220	
Coffee	10	280 Cal
SNACK		
Fresh fruit in season (peach, plum, etc)	70	
Coffee or tea	10	80 Cal
LUNCH		
Roast beef (2 oz) sandwich on whole-grain bread	295	
Lettuce	0	
Pickle spear	0	
Hot or iced tea	10	305 Cal
SNACK		
Coffee or tea	10	10 Cal
DINNER		
Frozen chicken dinner (Recipe 28 - page 104)	300	
Large tossed salad w 1½ Tbsp low-cal dressing	70	
Whole-grain bread (1 slice)	70	
Water	0	
Fiber One Chocolate Fudge Brownie	90	530 Cal
SNACK		
Coffee or tea	10	10 Cal
		1215 Cal

Day 29 Daily Menu

BREAKFAST	Calories	Totals
Orange juice (½ cup)	50	
Wild blueberry pancakes (Recipe 10 - page 86)	190	
Light syrup (1½ Tbsp)	45	
Coffee	10	295 Cal
SNACK		
Yogurt (6 oz nonfat, any flavor)	90	
Coffee or tea	10	100 Cal
LUNCH		
Salad (3 oz canned tuna, 1 tsp Evoo, onions, celery)	175	
Lettuce & tomato wedges	20	
Rye bread (1 slice)	70	
Fresh fruit in season (apple, pear, etc)	70	
Coffee or tea	10	345 Cal
SNACK		
Coffee or tea	10	10 Cal
DINNER		
Barbequed shrimp (Recipe 29 - page 105)	160	
Corn on the cob (medium)	90	
Steamed broccoli (1 cup – after cooking)	50	
Water	0	300 Cal
SNACK		
Kashi TLC Chewy Granola Bar	140	
Coffee or tea	10	150 Cal
		1200 Cal

Day 30 Daily Menu

BREAKFAST	Calories	Totals
Fresh orange sliced	75	
Kashi GoLean (1 cup) + ½ cup milk + ½ banana	235	
Coffee	10	320 Cal
SNACK		
Fresh fruit in season (apple, plum, etc)	70	
Coffee or tea	10	80 Cal
LUNCH		
Soup (Appendix B - page 137)	130	
Small whole-grain roll	80	
Raw zucchini slices, celery and carrot sticks	20	
Water	0	230 Cal
SNACK		
Coffee or tea	10	10 Cal
DINNER		
Cheeseburger (Recipe 30 - page 106)	370	
Lettuce and sliced tomato	20	
Whole-grain hard roll	140	
Steamed green beans	25	
Pickle spear	0	
Water	0	555 Cal
SNACK		
Coffee or tea	10	10 Cal
		1205 Cal

Day 31 Daily Menu

BREAKFAST	Calories	Totals
Grapefruit (½)	75	
Scrambled egg	80	
Whole grain toast (1 slice)	70	
Coffee	10	235 Cal
SNACK		
Yogurt (6 oz nonfat, any flavor)	90	
Coffee or tea	10	100 Cal
LUNCH		
Ham (2 oz) with mustard on 2 slices rye bread	300	
Pickle spear	0	
Hot or iced tea	10	310 Cal
SNACK		
Fresh fruit in season (apple, plum, etc)	70	
Coffee or tea	10	80 Cal
DINNER		
Baked Sea Bass (Recipe 31 - page 107)	395	
Large tossed salad w 1½ Tbsp low-cal dressing	70	
Water	0	465 Cal
SNACK		
Coffee or tea	10	10 Cal
		1200 Cal

Day 32 Daily Menu

BREAKFAST	Calories	Totals
Grapefruit (½)	75	
Cheerios (1 cup) + ½ cup skim milk + 15 raisins	190	
Coffee	10	275 Cal
SNACK		
Coffee or tea	10	10 Cal
LUNCH		
Subway 6" (Turkey Breast, Cheese + veggies)*	230	
Fresh fruit in season (apple, plum, etc)	70	
Coffee or tea	10	310 Cal
SNACK		
Handful unsalted mixed nuts	100	
Coffee or tea	10	110 Cal
DINNER		
Turkey tenders & veggies (Recipe 32 - page 108)	350	
Spinach (½ cup steamed drizzled w 1 tsp Evoo)	70	
Romaine lettuce, tomato w 1 Tbsp low-cal dressing	45	
Water with lemon wedge	10	475 Cal
SNACK		
Coffee or tea	10	10 Cal
* On 6" half wheat roll.		1190 Cal

Day 33 Daily Menu

BREAKFAST	Calories	Totals
Cantaloupe (½ medium)	50	
Fried egg	80	
Turkey bacon (1 slice)	35	
Toasted raisin bread (1 slice)	75	
Coffee	10	250 Cal
SNACK		
Yogurt (6 oz nonfat, any flavor)	90	
Coffee or tea	10	100 Cal
LUNCH		
Chicken, Broccoli & Cheddar*	270	
Hot or iced tea	10	280 Cal
* Hot Pockets wrap or an equivalent food.		
SNACK		
Coffee or tea	10	10 Cal
DINNER		
Frozen fish dinner (Recipe 33 - page 109)	340	
Large tossed salad w 1½ Tbsp low-cal dressing	70	
Whole-grain bread (1 slice)	70	
Fresh fruit in season (peach, plum, etc)	70	
Water	0	550 Cal
SNACK		
Coffee or tea	10	10 Cal
		1200 Cal

Day 34 Daily Menu

BREAKFAST	Calories	Totals
Tomato juice (½ cup)	20	
Shredded Wheat (1 cup) + ½ cup skim milk + ½ banana	265	
Coffee	10	295 Cal
SNACK		
Coffee or tea	10	10 Cal
LUNCH		
Roast beef (2 oz) with lettuce sandwich	300	
Hot or iced tea	10	310 Cal
SNACK		
Carrot sticks + ¼ cup low-fat cottage cheese & chives	60	
Coffee or tea	10	70 Cal
DINNER		
Pasta Rapini (Recipe 34 - page 110)	290	
Large tossed green salad with 1½ Tbsp low-cal	70	
Italian or French bread (1 slice)	80	
Water	0	440 Cal
SNACK		
Fresh fruit in season (apple, peach, etc)	70	
Coffee or tea	10	80 Cal
		1205 Cal

Day 35 Daily Menu

BREAKFAST	Calories	Totals
Cantaloupe (½ medium)	**50**	
Oatmeal ½ cup dry + ½ cup skim milk + about 15 raisins	**220**	
Coffee	**10**	**280 Cal**
## SNACK		
Fresh fruit in season (apple, plum, etc)	**70**	
Coffee or tea	**10**	**80 Cal**
## LUNCH		
Grilled cheese sandwich (2 slices 2% cheese)	**240**	
Pickle spear	**0**	
Water	**0**	**240 Cal**
## SNACK		
Carrot sticks + ¼ cup low-fat cottage cheese & chives	**60**	
Coffee or tea	**10**	**70 Cal**
## DINNER		
Eat Out – Chicken dinner (Recipe 35 - page 111)		
Max allowable calories	**530**	**530 Cal**
## SNACK		
Coffee or tea	**10**	**10 Cal**
		1210 Cal

Day 36 Daily Menu

BREAKFAST	Calories	Totals
Cantaloupe (½ medium)	50	
Wheaties (¾ cup) + ½ cup skim milk + ½ banana	190	
Coffee	10	250 Cal
SNACK		
Fresh fruit in season (apple, pear, etc)	70	
Coffee or tea	10	80 Cal
LUNCH		
Chorizo Egg & Cheese*	260	
Diet soda or water	0	260 Cal
* Hot Pockets wrap or an equivalent food.		
SNACK		
Coffee or tea	10	10 Cal
DINNER		
Grilled Tilapia (Recipe 36 - page 112)	300	
Asparagus spear (6)	25	
Wild rice (½ cup – after cooking)	100	
Large tossed salad with 1½ Tbsp low-cal dressing	70	
Water	0	495 Cal
SNACK		
Popcorn Mini Bag	110	
Coffee or tea	10	120 Cal
		1215 Cal

Day 37 Daily Menu

BREAKFAST	Calories	Totals
Orange juice (½ cup)	50	
Soft-boiled egg	80	
Whole grain toast (1 slice)	70	
Coffee	10	210 Cal
SNACK		
Yogurt (6 oz nonfat, any flavor)	90	
Coffee or tea	10	100 Cal
LUNCH		
Salad (3 oz canned tuna, 1 tsp Evoo, onions, celery)	175	
Lettuce & tomato wedges + rye bread (1 slice)	90	
Fresh fruit in season – (apple, pear, etc)	70	
Coffee or tea	10	345 Cal
SNACK		
Coffee or tea	10	10 Cal
DINNER		
Low-Cal Beef Stew (Recipe 37 - page 113)	365	
Large tossed salad with 1½ Tbsp low-cal dressing	70	
Small whole-grain roll	80	
Water with lemon wedge	10	525 Cal
SNACK		
Coffee or tea	10	10 Cal
		1200 Cal

Day 38 Daily Menu

BREAKFAST	Calories	Totals
Cantaloupe (½ medium)	50	
Smoothie (Recipe 14 - page 90)	220	
Coffee	10	280 Cal
SNACK		
Coffee or tea	10	10 Cal
LUNCH		
Peanut butter (2 Tbsp) on 2 slices whole-grain bread	340	
Skim milk (6 oz)	70	410 Cal
SNACK		
Fresh fruit in season (apple, plum, etc)	70	
Coffee or tea	10	80 Cal
DINNER		
Pan-broiled lamb chop (Recipe 38 - page 114)	320	
Large tossed salad with 1½ Tbsp low-cal dressing	70	
Water with lemon wedge	10	400 Cal
SNACK		
Coffee or tea	10	10 Cal
		1190 Cal

Day 39 Daily Menu

BREAKFAST	Calories	Totals
Fresh sliced orange	75	
Cheerios (1 cup) + ½ cup skim milk + about 15 raisins	190	
Coffee	10	275 Cal
SNACK		
Fresh fruit in season (peach, plum, etc)	70	
Coffee or tea	10	80 Cal
LUNCH		
Cottage cheese (1 cup low fat)	180	
Large tossed salad with 1½ Tbsp low-cal dressing	70	
Small whole-grain roll	80	
Hot or iced tea	10	340 Cal
SNACK		
Handful unsalted mixed nuts	100	
Coffee or tea	10	110 Cal
DINNER		
Chicken with veggies (Recipe 39 - page 115)	365	
Water with lemon wedge	10	375 Cal
SNACK		
Coffee or tea	10	10 Cal
		1190 Cal

Day 40 Daily Menu

BREAKFAST	Calories	Totals
Grapefruit (½)	75	
Scrambled egg	80	
Toasted raisin bread (1 slice)	75	
Coffee	10	240 Cal
SNACK		
Yogurt (6 oz nonfat, any flavor)	90	
Coffee or tea	10	100 Cal
LUNCH		
Soup (Appendix B - page 137)	170	
Whole-grain bread (1 slice)	70	
Hot or iced tea	10	250 Cal
SNACK		
Coffee or tea	10	10 Cal
DINNER		
Eat Out – Fish dinner (Recipe 40 - page 116)		
Max allowable calories	595	595 Cal
SNACK		
Coffee or tea	10	10 Cal
		1205 Cal

Day 41 Daily Menu

BREAKFAST	Calories	Totals
Orange juice (½ cup)	50	
Shredded Wheat (1 cup) + ½ cup skim milk + ½ banana	260	
Coffee	10	320 Cal
SNACK		
Coffee or tea	10	10 Cal
LUNCH		
Turkey frank (2 oz) with mustard & relish	150	
Hot dog bun	130	
Diet soda	0	280 Cal
SNACK		
Handful unsalted mixed nuts	100	
Coffee or tea	10	110 Cal
DINNER		
Pasta e Fagioli (Recipe 41 - page 117)	300	
Large tossed salad with 1½ Tbsp low-cal dressing	70	
Italian or French bread (1 slice)	80	
Water with lemon wedge	10	460 Cal
SNACK		
Coffee or tea	10	10 Cal
		1190 Cal

<u>Day 42 Daily Menu</u>

BREAKFAST	Calories	Totals
Cantaloupe (½ medium)	50	
Wheaties (¾ cup) + ½ cup skim milk + ½ banana	190	
Coffee	10	250 Cal
SNACK		
Coffee or tea	10	10 Cal
LUNCH		
Grilled Swiss cheese sandwich (2 oz low-fat cheese)	310	
Pickle spear	0	
Hot or iced tea	10	320 Cal
SNACK		
Fresh fruit in season (apple, peach, etc)	70	
Coffee or tea	10	80 Cal
DINNER		
Frozen chicken dinner (Recipe 28 - page 104)	300	
Large tossed salad with 1½ Tbsp low-cal dressing	70	
Water with lemon wedge	10	380 Cal
SNACK		
Blueberry Muffin (Recipe 42 - page 118)	145	
Coffee or tea	10	155 Cal
		1195 Cal

Day 43 Daily Menu

BREAKFAST	Calories	Totals
Fresh or frozen strawberries (½ cup)	25	
French toasted English Muffin Recipe 3 - page 79	270	
Light syrup (1 Tbsp)	30	
Coffee	10	335 Cal
SNACK		
Yogurt (6 oz nonfat, any flavor)	90	
Coffee or tea	10	100 Cal
LUNCH		
Salad (3 oz canned tuna, 1 tsp Evoo, onions, celery)	175	
Lettuce & tomato wedges	20	
Rye bread (1 slice)	70	
Coffee or tea	10	275 Cal
SNACK		
Coffee or tea	10	10 Cal
DINNER		
Beef Kebob with veggies (Recipe 43 - page 119)	390	
Baked potato (medium)	100	
Water	0	490 Cal
SNACK		
Coffee or tea	10	10 Cal
		1220 Cal

Day 44 Daily Menu

BREAKFAST	Calories	Totals
Orange juice (½ cup)	50	
Kashi GoLean (1 cup) + ½ cup skim milk + ½ banana	235	
Coffee	10	295 Cal
SNACK		
Coffee or tea	10	10 Cal
LUNCH		
Chicken, Broccoli & Cheddar*	270	
Diet soda or water	0	270 Cal
* Hot Pockets wrap or an equivalent food.		
SNACK		
Popcorn Mini Bag	110	
Coffee or tea	10	120 Cal
DINNER		
Baked Haddock (Recipe 44 - page 120)	420	
Large tossed salad with 1½ Tbsp low-cal dressing	70	
Water with lemon wedge	10	500 Cal
SNACK		
Coffee or tea	10	10 Cal
		1205 Cal

Day 45 Daily Menu

BREAKFAST	Calories	Totals
Cantaloupe (½ medium)	50	
Fried egg	80	
Toasted whole-grain bread (1 slice)	70	
Coffee	10	210 Cal
SNACK		
Yogurt (6 oz nonfat, any flavor)	90	
Coffee or tea	10	100 Cal
LUNCH		
Subway 6" (Ham, Cheese + veggies)*	260	
Large tossed salad with 1½ Tbsp low-cal dressing	70	
Hot or iced tea	10	340 Cal
SNACK		
Coffee or tea	10	10 Cal
DINNER		
Chicken Cacciatore (Recipe 45 - page 121)	310	
Italian or French bread (1 slice)	80	
Water	0	390 Cal
SNACK		
Blueberry muffin	145	
Coffee or tea	10	155 Cal
		1205 Cal

Day 46 Daily Menu

BREAKFAST	Calories	Totals
Grapefruit (½)	75	
Cheerios (1 cup) + ½ cup skim milk + about 15 raisins	190	
Coffee	10	275 Cal
SNACK		
Coffee or tea	10	10 Cal
LUNCH		
Cottage cheese (1 cup low fat)	180	
Large tossed salad with 1½ Tbsp low-cal dressing	70	
Hot or iced tea	10	260 Cal
SNACK		
Coffee or tea	10	10 Cal
DINNER		
Poached Cod (Recipe 46 - page 122)	275	
Grilled potatoes	100	
Grilled cherry tomatoes	45	
Spinach (½ cup) steamed with garlic & drizzled	50	
Water with lemon wedge	10	480 Cal
SNACK		
Blueberry muffin (See Recipe 42 - page 118)	145	
Coffee or tea	10	155 Cal
* On 6" half wheat roll.		1190 Cal

Day 47 Daily Menu

BREAKFAST	Calories	Totals
Grapefruit (½)	75	
Scrambled egg	80	
Whole-grain toast (1 slice)	70	
Coffee	10	235 Cal
SNACK		
Yogurt (6 oz nonfat, any flavor)	90	
Coffee or tea	10	100 Cal
LUNCH		
Soup (Appendix B - page 137)	90	
Turkey (1 oz) on 1 slice of rye bread (½ sandwich)	115	
Lettuce & tomato slices	20	
Water	0	225 Cal
SNACK		
Coffee or tea	10	10 Cal
DINNER		
Eat Out – Chinese food (Recipe 47 - page 123)		
Max allowable calories	640	640 Cal
SNACK		
Coffee or tea	10	10 Cal
		1220 Cal

<u>Day 48 Daily Menu</u>

BREAKFAST	Calories	Totals
Cantaloupe (½ medium)	50	
Smoothie (Recipe 14 - page 120)	220	
Coffee	10	280 Cal
<u>SNACK</u>		
Coffee or tea	10	10 Cal
<u>LUNCH</u>		
Left over Chinese food from Day 47	260	
Hot or iced tea	10	270 Cal
<u>SNACK</u>		
Coffee or tea	10	10 Cal
<u>DINNER</u>		
Healthy Pasta Salad (Recipe 48 - page 124)	370	
Italian or French bread (1 slice)	80	
Water with lemon wedge	10	460 Cal
<u>SNACK</u>		
Blueberry muffin	145	
Coffee or tea	10	155 Cal
		1185 Cal

Day 49 Daily Menu

BREAKFAST	Calories	Totals
Cantaloupe (½ medium)	50	
Oatmeal (½ cup dry) + ½ cup milk + about 15 raisins	220	
Coffee	10	280 Cal
SNACK		
Coffee or tea	10	10 Cal
LUNCH		
Turkey breast (2 oz) on 2 slices whole-grain bread	245	
Lettuce, tomato and 1 Tbsp light mayo	35	
Pickle spear	0	
Water with lemon wedge	10	290 Cal
SNACK		
Fresh fruit in season (apple, plum, etc)	70	
Coffee or tea	10	80 Cal
DINNER		
Frozen meat dinner (Recipe 21 - page 125)	300	
Large tossed salad with 1½ Tbsp low-cal dressing	70	
Water with lemon wedge	10	380 Cal
SNACK		
Blueberry muffin	145	
Coffee or tea	10	155 Cal
		1195 Cal

Day 50 Daily Menu

BREAKFAST	Calories	Totals
Fresh or frozen strawberries (1 cup)	25	
French toasted English Muffin (Recipe 3 - page 79)	270	
Light syrup (1 Tbsp)	30	
Coffee	10	335 Cal
SNACK		
Yogurt (6 oz nonfat, any flavor)	90	
Coffee or tea	10	100 Cal
LUNCH		
Soup (Appendix B - page 137)	100	
BLT sandwich - 2 slices turkey bacon, 1 Tbsp light mayo	245	
Pickle spear	0	
Hot or iced tea	10	355 Cal
SNACK		
Coffee or tea	10	10 Cal
DINNER		
Pan-fried Sole (Recipe 50 - page 126)	325	
Large tossed salad with 1½ Tbsp low-cal dressing	70	
Water	0	395 Cal
SNACK		
Coffee or tea	10	10 Cal
		1205 Cal

<h1 align="center">Day 51 Daily Menu</h1>

BREAKFAST	Calories	Totals
Cantaloupe (½ medium)	50	
Wheaties (¾ cup) + ½ cup skim milk + ½ banana	190	
Coffee	10	250 Cal
SNACK		
Coffee or tea	10	10 Cal
LUNCH		
Ham (2 oz) with mustard on 2 slices rye bread	290	
Pickle spear	0	
Hot or iced tea	10	300 Cal
SNACK		
Handful unsalted mixed nuts	100	
Coffee or tea	10	110 Cal
DINNER		
Beans and Greens Salad (Recipe 51 - page 127)	260	
Whole-grain bread (1 slice)	70	
Baked potato (medium)	100	
Water with lemon wedge	10	510 Cal
SNACK		
Coffee or tea	10	10 Cal
		1190 Cal

Day 52 Daily Menu

BREAKFAST	Calories	Totals
Fresh orange sliced	75	
Soft-boiled egg	80	
Whole-grain toast (1 slice)	70	
Coffee	10	235 Cal
SNACK		
Coffee or tea	10	10 Cal
LUNCH		
Salad – 3 oz canned salmon, 1 tsp Evoo, onions & celery	200	
Lettuce & tomato wedges	20	
Rye bread (1 slice)	70	
Water	0	290 Cal
SNACK		
Fresh fruit in season (apple, plum, etc)	70	
Coffee or tea	10	80 Cal
DINNER		
Chicken Piccata (Recipe 52 - page 128)	270	
Brown rice (½ cup – after cooking)	100	
Large tossed salad with 1½ Tbsp low-cal dressing	70	
Water	10	450 Cal
SNACK		
Graham crackers (3 squares)	90	
Skim milk (4 oz)	45	135 Cal
		1200 Cal

Day 53 Daily Menu

BREAKFAST	Calories	Totals
Grapefruit (½)	75	
Cheerios (1 cup) + ½ cup skim milk + about 15 raisins	190	
Coffee	10	275 Cal
SNACK		
Fresh fruit in season (peach, plum, etc)	70	
Coffee or tea	10	80 Cal
LUNCH		
Cottage cheese (1 cup low fat)	180	
Large tossed salad with 1½ Tbsp low-cal dressing	70	
Hot or iced tea	10	260 Cal
SNACK		
Handful unsalted mixed nuts	100	
Coffee or tea	10	110 Cal
DINNER		
Beef steak strips (Recipe 53 - page 129)	330	
Steamed spinach (½ cup)	25	
Baked potato (medium)	100	
Water with lemon wedge	10	465 Cal
SNACK		
Coffee or tea	10	10 Cal
		1200 Cal

<h1 style="text-align:center"><u>Day 54 Daily Menu</u></h1>

BREAKFAST	Calories	Totals
Cantaloupe (½ medium)	50	
Fried egg	80	
Toasted whole-grain bread (1 slice)	70	
Coffee	10	210 Cal
SNACK		
Coffee or tea	10	10 Cal
LUNCH		
Soup (Appendix B - page 137)	200	
Hard whole-grain roll (medium)	80	
Lettuce & tomato slices	20	
Water	0	300 Cal
SNACK		
Fresh fruit in season (apple, peach, etc)	70	
Coffee or tea	10	80 Cal
DINNER		
Grilled scallops (Recipe 54 - page 130)	210	
Grilled polenta (Recipe 54)	125	
Mushroom-steamed green beans-red onion (Recipe 54)	45	
Grilled asparagus (Recipe 54)	10	
Large tossed salad with 1½ Tbsp low-cal dressing	70	
Water	0	460 Cal
SNACK		
Graham crackers (2 squares)	60	
Skim milk (6 oz)	70	130 Cal
		1190 Cal

<h1 style="text-align:center"><u>Day 55 Daily Menu</u></h1>

BREAKFAST	Calories	Totals
Cantaloupe (½ medium)	**50**	
Oatmeal (½ cup dry) + ½ cup skim milk + about 15 raisins	**220**	
Coffee	**10**	**280 Cal**
SNACK		
Coffee or tea	**10**	**10 Cal**
LUNCH		
Left over Bean Salad from Day 23 (1 serving)	**260**	
Small whole-grain roll	**80**	
Lettuce & tomato slices	**20**	
Hot or iced tea	**10**	**370 Cal**
SNACK		
Coffee or tea	**10**	**10 Cal**
DINNER		
Hearty Vegetable Soup (Recipe 55 - page 13)	**360**	
Large tossed salad with 1½ Tbsp low-cal dressing	**70**	
Italian or French bread (1 slice)	**80**	
Water	**0**	**510 Cal**
SNACK		
Coffee or tea	**10**	**10 Cal**
		1190 Cal

<u>Day 56 Daily Menu</u>

BREAKFAST	Calories	Totals
Tomato juice (½ cup)	20	
Shredded Wheat (1 cup) + ½ cup skim milk + ½ banana	260	
Coffee	10	290 Cal
SNACK		
Coffee or tea	10	10 Cal
LUNCH		
Roast beef (2 oz) sandwich on whole-grain bread	305	
Lettuce	0	
Fresh fruit in season (pear, plum, etc)	70	
Water	0	375 Cal
SNACK		
Carrot sticks + ¼ cup low-fat cottage cheese & chives	60	
Coffee or tea	10	70 Cal
DINNER		
Frozen chicken dinner (Recipe 56 - page 132)	300	
Large tossed salad with 1½ Tbsp low-cal dressing	70	
Whole-grain bread (1 slice)	70	
Water	0	440 Cal
SNACK		
Coffee or tea	10	10 Cal
		1195 Cal

Day 57 Daily Menu

BREAKFAST	Calories	Totals
Cantaloupe (½ medium)	50	
Smoothie (Recipe 14 - page 90)	220	
Coffee	10	280 Cal
SNACK		
Coffee or tea	10	10 Cal
LUNCH		
Salad (3 oz canned tuna, 1 tsp Evoo, onions, celery)	175	
Lettuce & tomato wedges	20	
Rye bread (1 slice)	70	
Fresh fruit in season (apple, pear, etc)	70	
Coffee or tea	10	345 Cal
SNACK		
Coffee or tea	10	10 Cal
DINNER		
Salmon with Mango Salsa (Recipe 57 - page 133)	460	
Large tossed salad with 1½ Tbsp low-cal dressing	70	
Water with lemon wedge	10	540 Cal
SNACK		
Coffee or tea	10	10 Cal
		1195 Cal

Day 58 Daily Menu

BREAKFAST	Calories	Totals
Tomato juice (½ cup)	20	
Kashi GoLean (1 cup) + ½ cup skim milk + ½ banana	235	
Coffee	10	265 Cal
SNACK		
Coffee or tea	10	10 Cal
LUNCH		
Soup (Appendix B - page 137)	120	
Small whole-grain roll	80	
Hot or iced tea	10	200 Cal
SNACK		
Coffee or tea	10	10 Cal
DINNER		
Grilled pork chop with orange (Recipe 58 - page 134)	470	
Wild rice (¼ cup – after cooking)	50	
Asparagus (7 spear cooked & drained)	20	
Water with lemon wedge	10	550 Cal
SNACK		
Blueberry muffin	145	
Coffee or tea	10	155 Cal
		1200 Cal

Day 59 Daily Menu

BREAKFAST	Calories	Totals
Grapefruit (½)	75	
Scrambled egg	80	
Whole-grain toast (1 slice)	70	
Coffee	10	235 Cal
SNACK		
Yogurt (6 oz nonfat, any flavor)	90	
Coffee or tea	10	100 Cal
LUNCH		
Soup (Appendix B - page 137)	120	
Tomato slices ¼ cup chopped fresh basil + 1 tsp Evoo	60	
Whole-grain bread (1 slice)	70	
Hot or iced tea	10	260 Cal
SNACK		
Coffee or tea	10	10 Cal
DINNER		
Eat Out – Fish dinner (Recipe 59 - page 135)		
Max allowable calories	595	595 Cal
SNACK		
Coffee or tea	10	10 Cal
		1210 Cal

Day 60 Daily Menu

BREAKFAST	Calories	Totals
Grapefruit (½)	75	
Cheerios (1 cup) + ½ cup skim milk + about 15 raisins	190	
Coffee	10	275 Cal
SNACK		
Coffee or tea	10	10 Cal
LUNCH		
Subway 6" (Ham, Cheese + veggies)*	260	
Water (or diet soda)	0	260 Cal
SNACK		
Handful unsalted mixed nuts	100	
Coffee or tea	10	110 Cal
DINNER		
Chicken Stew (Recipe 60 - page 136)	360	
Brown rice (½ cup – after cooking)	100	
Small whole-grain roll	80	
Water	0	540 Cal
SNACK		
Coffee or tea	10	10 Cal
* On 6" half wheat roll.		1205 Cal

Day 1- Recipe

Chicken with Peppers & Onions

   4 boneless and skinless chicken breasts (about 5 oz each)
Coat the chicken breasts in a bottled barbeque sauce. Prepare medium-hot fire on well-oiled grill. Place breasts on grill, turning them every 4 minutes, for 10 to 12 minutes, or until done. (To check if breasts are done, the meat should be moist and white with no sign of pink when you cut into the breast.) Salt and pepper to taste.

   2 medium red peppers, sliced
   1 medium onion, sliced
Place peppers and onions in pan with 2 tablespoons fat-free chicken stock. Sauté until stock is reduced. Spray pan lightly with non-stick cooking oil and cook another 2 minutes. Salt and pepper to taste.
Serves 4. About 250 Calories per serving (for chicken only).

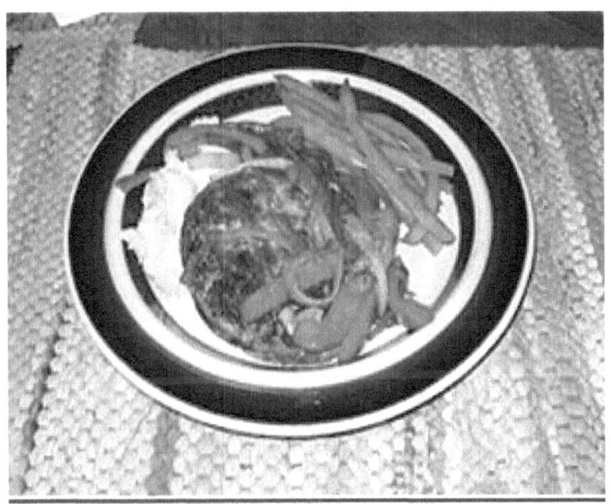

Diet Tip of the Day: Weight Loss – take it one step, one meal, one workout, one day at a time. Just think of where you'll be in 90 days!

Day 2 - Recipe

Baked Herb-Crusted Cod

4 cod fish fillets (4 to 5 ounces each)
2 tablespoons flour
2 tablespoons cornmeal
2 tablespoons minced fresh herbs
2 teaspoons lemon juice

Sprinkle cod with lemon juice. Mix flour, cornmeal and herbs and dust the cod with the cornmeal-herb mixture. Bake in oven at 375 °F for 10 minutes. Add salt and black pepper to taste.

Serves 4. One serving is about 230 Calories (for cod only).

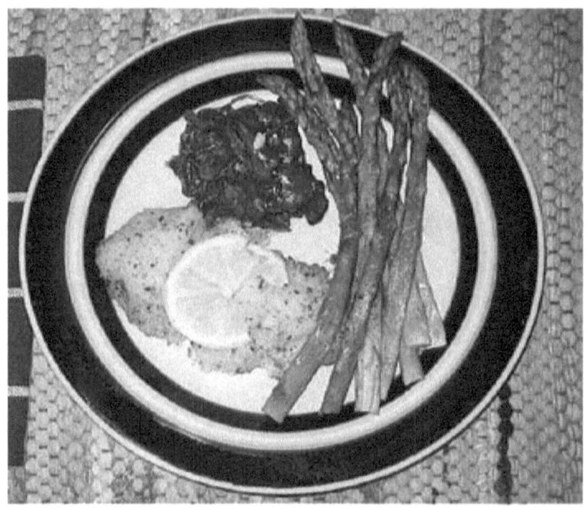

Diet Tip of the Day:. A **reducing diet is best supervised by a physician**. This is especially true when a great deal of weight needs to be lost, or if you have an ailment or a history of medical problems.

Day 3 - Recipe

French-Toasted English Muffin

    6 whole wheat light English muffins, sliced in half
    4 eggs
    2 cups skim milk
    2 teaspoons vanilla
    A dash of cinnamon

In a medium bowl, beat together eggs and skim milk. Add vanilla and cinnamon. Slice English muffins into halves and saturate slices in egg mixture. In a non-stick skillet coated with cooking spray, cook muffins until both sides are golden brown. Dust lightly with confectionary sugar. Serve hot or keep in an oven or warmer at 200 ºF until ready to plate. **Serves 4**. Three English muffin slices per serving. Serving is 270 Calories.

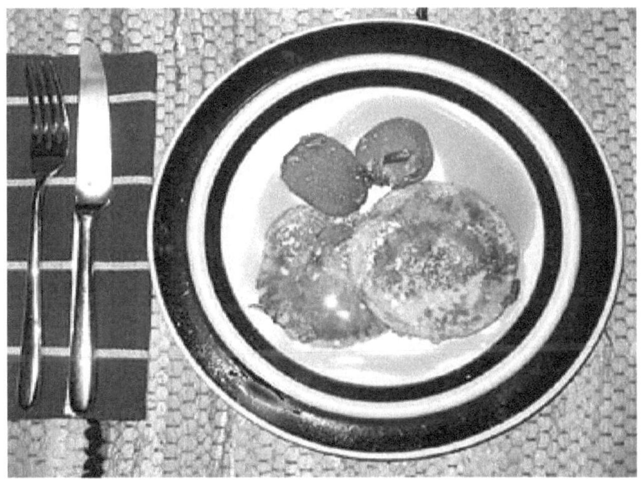

Diet Tip of the Day: **"Eat Slowly"** This is especially vital when you are trying to lose weight. If you are someone who eats fast, who finishes before everyone else at the table, you are not giving yourself a chance to feel full. While everyone else is still eating, you either sit there and pick, or you have seconds, taking in extra calories you could avoid if you would just slow down.

Day 4 - Recipe

<u>Carrie's Low-Cal Meat Loaf</u>

½ pound ground white meat turkey
½ pound ground beef (about 90% lean)
1 large egg
½ cup skim milk
¼ cup bread crumbs
¼ cup ketchup
¼ cup chopped carrots
¼ cup chopped onion

In a medium bowl, combine all ingredients. Add salt and pepper to taste. Mix until blended and form into a loaf. Place loaf into oven preheated to 350 °F. Bake until an instant-read thermometer inserted in the center of the loaf reads 160 °F. This should take about one hour.

Shown below is meat loaf, acorn squash (baked with 1 teaspoon of maple syrup). Also shown is steamed spinach drizzled with extra-virgin olive oil.

<u>Serves 5</u>. About 290 Calories per serving (for meat loaf only). Note: reserve half a serving of the meat loaf which is to be eaten for lunch on Day 6.

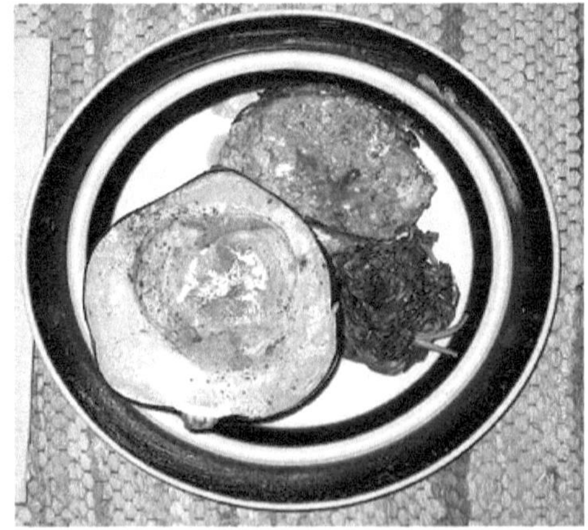

<u>**Diet Tip of the Day:**</u> **Take a daily multi-vitamin/mineral supplement.** This is very important when you're on a diet – as a kind of insurance policy.

Day 5 - Recipe

<u>Frozen-Fish Dinner</u>

No recipe today. No cooking today. It's your day off! Some reasonably good frozen fish dinners are:

Shrimp Alfredo	**Lean Cuisine**	~~230~~ 240
Tuna Noodle Casserole	**Smart Ones**	~~250~~ 270
Shrimp & Angel Hair Pasta	**Lean Cuisine**	~~280~~ 290
Parmesan Crusted Fish	**Lean Cuisine**	~~290~~ 300
Tortilla Crusted Fish	**Lean Cuisine**	~~300~~ 310

That's it. At this writing, there are just not that many frozen fish dinners for sale at supermarkets, although new entrees are being introduced continually. If you choose any of the above entrees, you will not use all of the **340 Calories allocated for this meal**. In this case, use the excess calories anyway you wish. Splurge on extra dessert or save the calories for another day!

See **Appendix B** on page 138 for our comprehensive list of frozen entrees. Please read the important **Frozen-Food Safety Warning** in **Appendix C** on page 143.

<u>Diet Tip of the Day:</u> **Buy a pedometer** and start walking. For the average person 2100 steps amounts to walking about one mile. A Harvard study has shown that 8000 to 10,000 step per day promote weight loss. And you're not obliged to walk continuously until you accrue all 10,000 steps. Rather, all steps throughout the day to wherever and whenever count toward your daily total. Because 10,000 steps a day may not be achievable by some people, particularly those who are elderly, sedentary, or who have chronic diseases, rather than insisting on a blanket 10,000 steps per day, your initial stepping goal should your baseline steps plus an increment of an additional 2500 steps . (Your baseline being the number of steps you take in an average day.)

81

Day 6 - Recipe

Grandma's Pizza

The following is a pizza recipe used by Gail Johnson's Italian grandmother. She was from a small mountain village located between Rome and Naples.

Pizza dough: To save time use prepared dough, preferably whole wheat. To start, flour a large cutting board. Divide one pound of prepared pizza dough into four parts. Roll out each dough ball as thin as possible.

Tomato sauce: Sauté ½ small onion, chopped fine, in 1 teaspoon olive oil. Add two finely chopped garlic cloves, 1½ cups chopped plum tomatoes and ½ teaspoon chopped fresh oregano. Stir and cook about 5 minutes on a low flame.

Pizza preparation & cooking: On each pizza, spread evenly ¼ cup of the tomato sauce. Add ½ ounce of shredded part-skim mozzarella cheese, 1 teaspoon Parmesan cheese, 3 slices of a Portobello mushroom, some torn fresh basil, and drizzle with extra-virgin olive oil. Put pizzas on a pan and place in 475 °F oven for about 15 to 20 minutes, or until crust is crisp and cheese is just melting. (Freeze left over sauce for use on Day 13.)

<u>Serves 4</u>. Each pizza contains approximately 350 Calories.

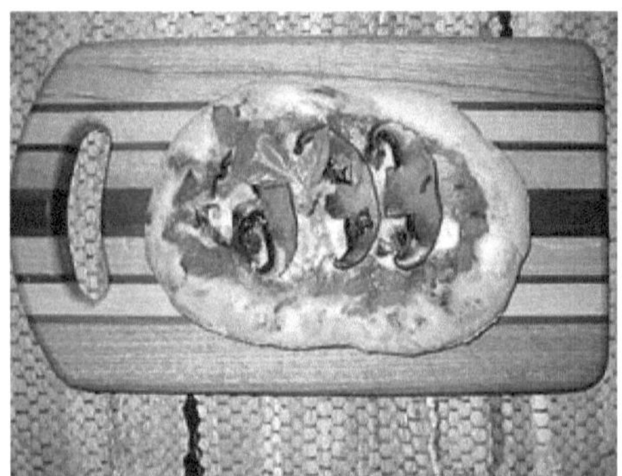

<u>Diet Tip of the Day:</u> For **life-long weight control** take a vigorous 30 to 60 minute walk everyday! That's right – everyday. Make exercise a nonflexible top priority part of your life. When it comes to exercise the key words are consistent, persistent, unyielding, dogged. Get the point?

Day 7 - Recipe

<u>Chicken Dinner - Out</u>

No recipe today. No cooking today. Have a chicken dinner at your
favorite restaurant, but make sure you choose a restaurant where you
have a fighting chance to achieve your calorie goal. For your chicken
dinner out, your maximum allowable calories (includes appetizer, soup,
main course and dessert) are as follows:

- For the **1200 Calorie Diet**: 530 Calories
- For the **1500 Calorie Diet**: 630 Calories
- For the **1800 Calorie Diet**: 630 Calories

Tips for Eating Chicken Out: First, order simple and order skinless
white meat only, such as broiled chicken breast with steamed vegetables
and brown rice. Tell the waiter you want no sauce, no gravy, nothing
added. Then, knowing your calorie objective, and that chicken is about
50 Calories per ounce, most steamed vegetable servings average
approximately 50 Calories per cup, and rice is about 100 Calories per ½
cup, decide how much to eat – and take the remainder home. If fresh
fruit is not an option, pass on dessert and have the evening snack
specified for that day in this diet.

In a restaurant, most nutritionists recommend you eat the low-
calorie items on your plate first. Start with the salad, soup and veggies.
By the time you get to the chicken and starches you will hopefully be full
enough to be content with smaller portions of the higher-calorie choices.
(Incidentally, feel free to substitute skinless white meat turkey for
chicken.)

Finally, some dieticians advise their dieting clients not to eat out.
That's right. They believe eating at home is safer. But our thought is
you have to eat out eventually so why not learn how while your resolve
is high?

<u>Diet Tip of the Day:</u> When you're on a diet, eating in a restaurant can
be a challenge, because most restaurant portions are huge, and can easily
total more than 1000 Calories. So, in a restaurant decide how much to eat
– and take the remainder home. A good general rule of thumb is to **eat
half and bring the rest home**.

Day 8 - Recipe

Baked Salmon with Salsa

This is a simple, straight-forward recipe. The advantage of a simple recipe is there are no hidden calories.

4   5 oz salmon fillets
6   tablespoons bottled tomato-pepper salsa

Brown salmon fillets in non-stick pan and then place them in a baking dish. Cook fillets in an oven preheated to 350 °F for about 10 minutes. Plate the salmon. Stir bottled tomato-pepper salsa and spoon it over the salmon.

Serves 4. One salmon fillet is about 215 Calories.

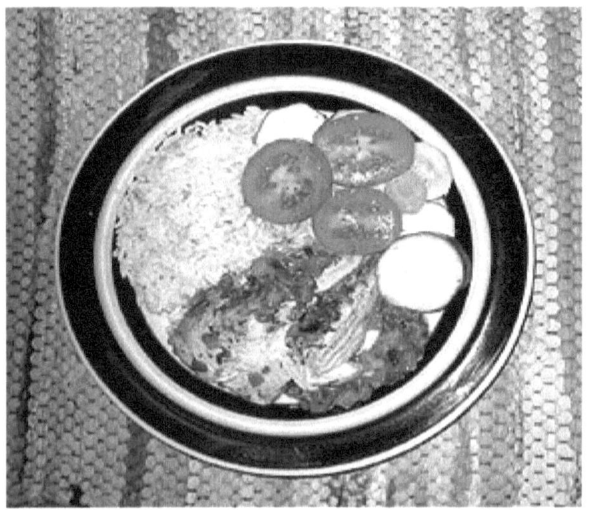

Diet Tip of the Day: Hunger is your body's way of telling you that you need calories. But **when you're done eating, you should feel better – satisfied but not stuffed**.

Day 9 - Recipe

Veggie Burger

Vegetable-based burgers can be purchased at your local supermarket. Patties of a veggie burger are made from either vegetables, soy, nuts, mushrooms, textured vegetable protein, dairy, or a combination of these foods.

In the U.S., two popular veggie burgers are the Boca Burger and Gardenburger. The Boca Burger is made chiefly from soy protein and wheat gluten. (Boca Burger patties are 2.5 oz each and range from 60 to 90 Calories.) The original Gardenburger is made from mushrooms, onions, brown rice, rolled oats, cheese, and spices. (Gardenburger patties are 2.5 oz each and about 100 Calories.)

To prepare, follow package directions. The version shown below has an added slice of low-fat cheddar cheese. The lettuce, tomato and ketchup shown actually add very few extra calories.

The veggie burger patty plus low-fat cheese amounts to approximately 150 Calories. Add a seeded roll and the total rises to 290 Calories.

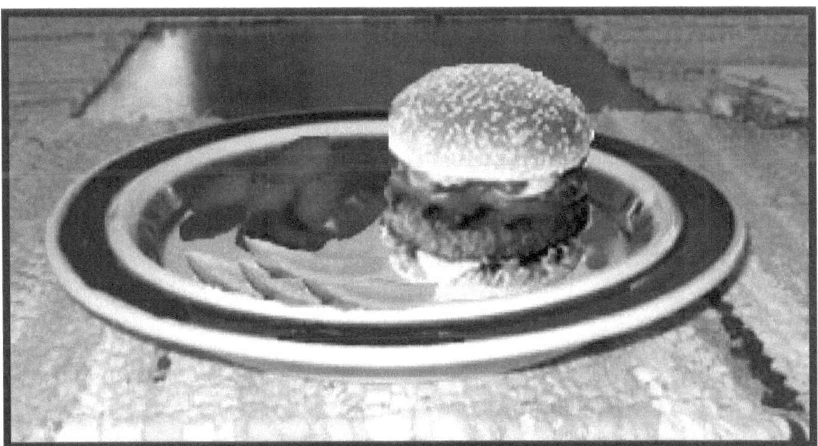

<u>**Diet Tip of the Day:**</u> **Drink lots of water** – about 8 glasses per day when you're trying to lose weight. Add a slice of lemon to make it more interesting. Often, when you think you're hungry, you are just thirsty. So, next time you crave a snack, drink some water first and see if that does it for you.

Day 10 - Recipe

<u>Wild Blueberry Pancakes</u>

This recipe makes a relatively low calorie, wholesome batch of delicious wild blueberry-whole wheat-buttermilk pancakes.

1 cup whole-wheat flour

1 cup buttermilk

1 egg

1 tablespoon vegetable oil

1 teaspoon baking powder

½ teaspoon baking soda

Stir ingredients until blended. Add ¾ cup fresh of frozen blueberries and gently stir. Using medium heat, preheat a non-stick skillet coated with cooking spray. Pour slightly less than ¼ cup of batter onto skillet per pancake. Cook slowly until bubbles break on surface of pancake. Turn and cook until other side is lightly browned.

Makes 8 pancakes. Pictured below are wild-blueberry pancakes with two slices of turkey bacon.

<u>Serves 4</u>. Each pancake is about 95 Calories

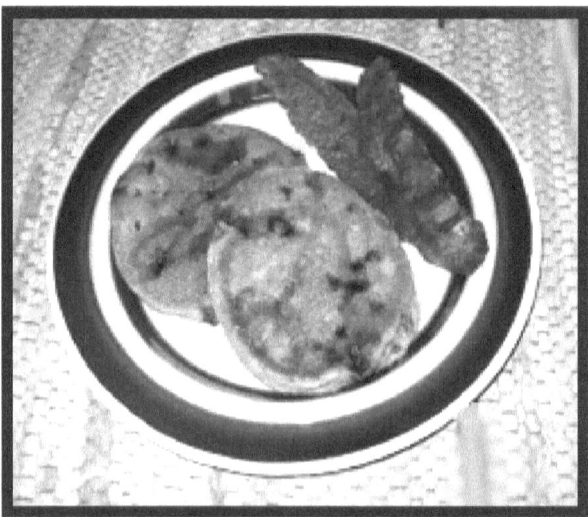

Bacon allowable only on 1500 and 1800 Calorie diets.

<u>**Diet Tip of the Day:**</u> Most experts associate eating a substantial breakfast with successful weight loss.

<h1>Day 11 - Recipe</h1>

Artichoke-Bean Salad

19-ounce can white kidney beans
10 artichoke hearts, quartered
⅓ cup chopped oregano
⅓ cup chopped parsley
3 cloves garlic, chopped
1 lemon, juiced

Combine ingredients in medium-size bowl. Stir in ¼ cup extra-virgin olive oil. Salt and black pepper to taste.

Serves 6. Approximately 190 Calories per serving.

Pictured on the plate below is the <u>artichoke-bean salad</u> as a side dish with two grilled chicken sausage links, tomato salsa and steamed green beans. Incidentally, this artichoke-bean combination over mixed salad greens served with a whole-grain bread makes a delicious, nutritious and reasonable low-calorie main course.

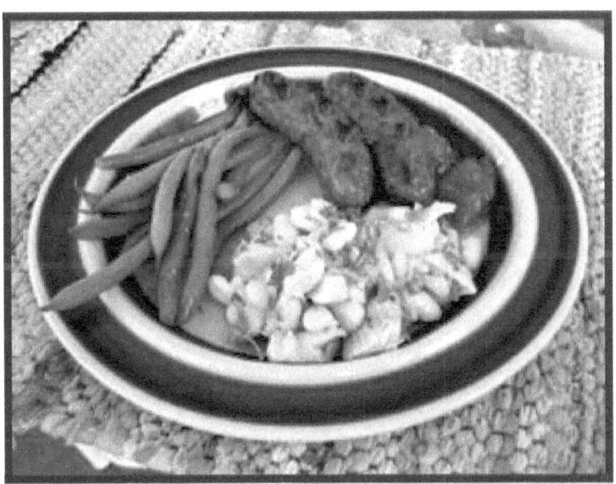

Diet Tip of the Day: Before you go to a **party**, have a small meal, such as a hardboiled egg, an apple, and a thirst quencher (like water, tea, seltzer, or diet soda). This will take the edge off your appetite and make it easier to resist the high-calorie goodies.

<u>Day 12 - Recipe</u>

<u>Fish Dinner - Out</u>

No recipe today. No cooking today. Have a fish dinner at your favorite restaurant, but make sure you choose a restaurant where you have a good chance to achieve your calorie goal. For today, your **goal for dinner is a maximum of 595 Calories**. This includes appetizer, soup, main course and dessert.

     Tips for Eating Fish Out: The following is almost an exact repeat of the advice given eating out on previous days. First, order simple, such as broiled fish with steamed vegetables and brown rice. Tell the waiter you want no sauce, no gravy, nothing added. Then, knowing your calorie objective, and that fish is about 50 Calories per ounce, most steamed vegetable servings average approximately 50 Calories per cup, and rice is about 100 Calories per ½ cup, decide how much to eat – and take the remainder home. If fresh fruit is not an option, pass on dessert and have the evening snack specified for that day in the diet.

     In a restaurant, some nutritionists recommend you eat the low-calorie items on your plate first. Start with the salad, soup and veggies. By the time you get to the fish and starches you will hopefully be full enough to be content with smaller portions of the higher-calorie choices.

<u>**Diet Tip of the Day:**</u> Phytonutrients are found in plant foods such as fruits, vegetables, whole grains, dried beans, nuts and seeds. Unlike protein, fat, vitamins and minerals, phytonutrients are not necessary for life, but evidence is growing that phytonutrients have many beneficial qualities.

Day 13 - Recipe

Pasta with Marinara Sauce

Prepare the sauce as you did for the Day 6 pizza (on page 112). But because the pizza sauce is a bit too thick, we add ¼ cup of pasta liquid to thin it. (The spiral pasta profile shown below is called fusilli, a very popular pasta shape because all those ridges hold buckets of tomato sauce.)

   ½ pound <u>whole-wheat</u> pasta
   ¼ teaspoon salt

Prepare the marinara tomato sauce as per Day 6 sauce but dilute it with ¼ cup of today's pasta liquid.

Bring 2 quarts of lightly salted water to a boil. Add pasta and stir occasionally (to keep pasta from sticking to the bottom of the pot). Keep water boiling and cook until pasta are "al dente." (Cooking time is approximately 9 minutes.) Drain pasta, add marinara sauce and serve hot.

Serves 4. One serving is about 225 Calories.

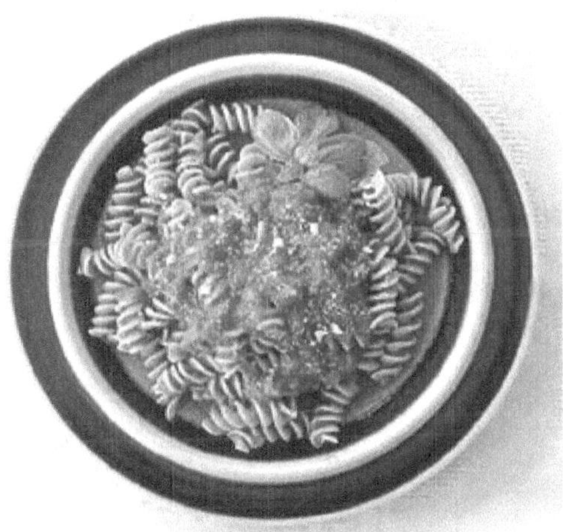

Diet Tip of the Day: **Beware of alcoholic beverages**. Beer has about 13 Calories per ounce, wine 25 Calories per ounce and whiskey a whopping 71 Calories per ounce.

Day 14 - Recipe

<u>Low-Cal Smoothie</u>

Smoothies are delicious, nutritious and fun to drink! They're great for a fast but nutritious breakfast, a light energy-boosting lunch, a healthy snack, a late afternoon pick me up, and a delicious dessert. Making your own smoothie is a smart way to save money and get healthy at the same time!

8 ounces plain fat-free yogurt

1 cup orange juice

1 cup strawberries

½ cup blueberries

1 banana

1 teaspoon sugar

1 teaspoon vanilla extract

Place yogurt, strawberries, and blueberries in a blender. Pour in orange juice. Add sugar and vanilla extract to mixture. Blend all ingredients until thick and smooth. Pour smoothie into a glass and enjoy.

<u>Serves 2</u>. About 220 Calories per serving

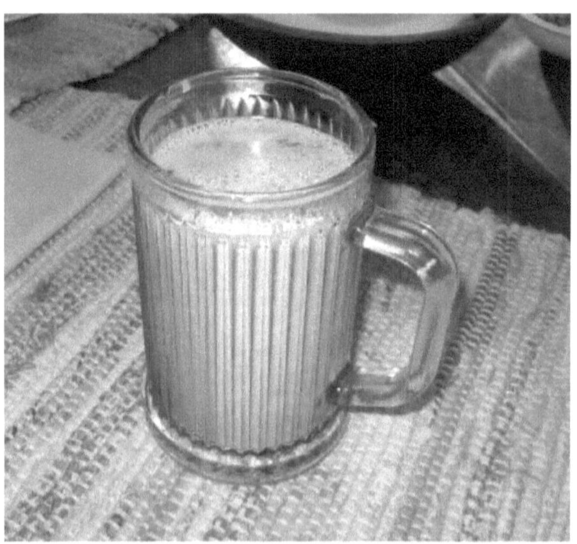

<u>Diet Tip of the Day:</u> Two scientific journals indicate **dark chocolate** - not white chocolate or milk chocolate - is potent antioxidant and is good for you. But don't overdo it, because you have to offset the extra chocolate calories by eating less of other foods.

<h1 style="text-align:center">Day 15 - Recipe</h1>

<u>London Broil</u>

   1 lb boneless flank steak about ¾" thick, fat trimmed
   1 clove garlic
   1 teaspoon dry oregano

Rub each side of the flank steak with garlic. Season with oregano, salt and pepper to taste. Prepare a large non-stick skillet over high heat. Steak should sizzle when placed on hot skillet. Sear steak on one side for about 5 minutes; then turn and sear other side for about 4 minutes, or until done to preference. Check the center by making small incision. Carve into ¼-inch slices.

<u>Serves 4</u>. About 320 Calories per serving (for meat only).

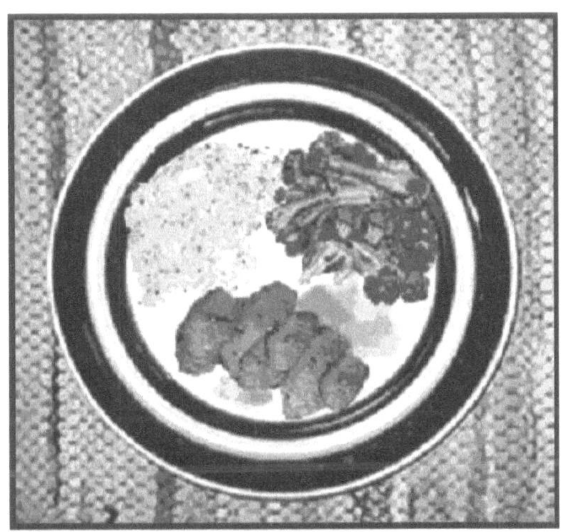

<u>Diet Tip of the Day:</u> **Stay Busy.** Most people will do anything to avoid work, housework, yard work, exercise, etc. But any kind of work burns a lot more calories than just sitting! Whatever it is you are avoiding – just go do it!

Day 16 - Recipe
<u>Red Snapper with Special Sauce</u>

    4 4-ounce red snapper fillets (salmon fillets okay)
    ½ cup white wine
    ½ cup non-fat yogurt mixed with ¼ cup mustard
    ½ pound green beans
    ¾ pint cherry tomatoes (about 20), halved
    4 teaspoons olive oil
    ¾ cup wild rice, brown rice and wheat berry mix.

Brown fillets in non-stick pan. Place fillets skin side down in baking dish coated with non-stick spray. Add white wine and cook in oven preheated to 350 °F for about 15 minutes . Spoon pan juices over fillets. Salt and pepper to taste.

Place green beans in skillet. Add ¼-inch of water and cook over medium heat until water boils off. Add cherry tomatoes and olive oil. Stir well and sauté for a few minutes. (If desired, season with fresh rosemary and oregano.) Salt and pepper to taste.

Prepare rice mix per package directions.

Plate red snapper fillet and spoon over yogurt-mustard sauce. Add green beans and tomato mix and the wild rice mix. Serve hot.
<u>Serves 4.</u> One plate consisting of a snapper fillet (215 Cal) with green beans & tomato mix (75 Cal) and wild rice (160 Cal) totals 450 Calories.

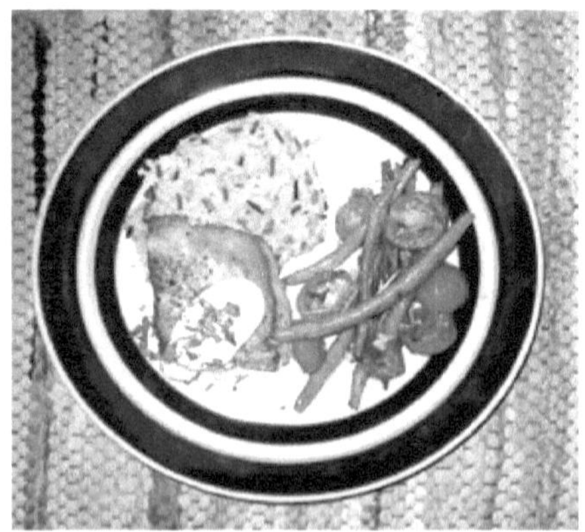

<u>Diet Tip of the Day:</u> **Don't have sweets in your house**. This makes them easier to resist. Out of sight, out of mind!

Day 17 - Recipe

Cajun Chicken Salad

This is a perfect after-work, quick, nutritious and delicious dinner.

    4 boneless and skinless chicken breasts - about 5 oz each
    4 teaspoons of bottled Cajun herb-spice mix
    8 ounces mixed salad greens
    ¾ pint cherry tomatoes (about 20), halved
    12 pitted black olives
    2 tablespoons bottled light salad dressing

Brush chicken breasts lightly with olive oil. Roll breasts in Cajun herb-spice mix.

Brown breasts on non-stick oven-proof skillet. After breasts are brown, put skillet in 350 °F oven for approximately 15 minutes, or until done. (When the breasts are done, the meat should be moist and white with no sign of pink.) Cut breasts into ½-inch slices.

Serve hot or keep in an oven or warmer at 200 °F until ready to plate. Place chicken slices over a bed of mixed salad greens. Add tomatoes, olives and two tablespoons of your favorite low-calorie salad dressing. **Serves 4**. 330 Calories per serving

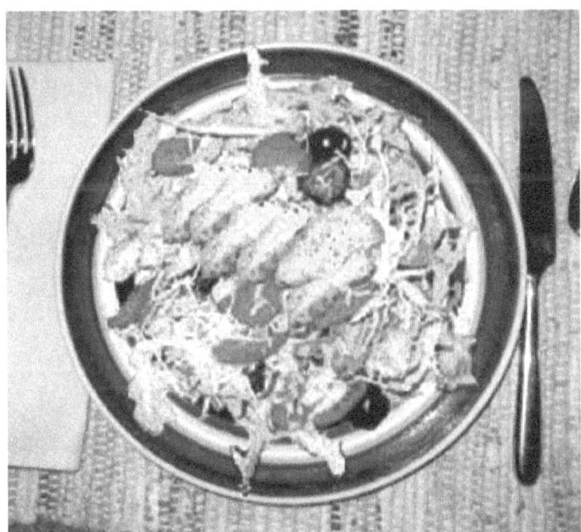

Diet Tip of the Day: Hot or cold cereal topped with fruit, and fat-free milk makes a nutritious, relatively low-calorie meal anytime.

Day 18 - Recipe

Grilled Swordfish

1¼ pounds swordfish
1 bottle citrus-herb marinade
¾ pint cherry tomatoes (about 20), halved
4 medium potatoes
2 cups fresh spinach
1 teaspoon rosemary & juice of ¼ lemon
2 teaspoon extra-virgin olive oil, divided
Steam spinach with garlic and drizzle with about 1 teaspoon extra-virgin olive oil.

Cut potatoes in medium-size pieces and sprinkle with lemon juice, add rosemary, salt and black pepper. Place potatoes on grill for about 10 minutes, turning occasionally.

Toss cherry tomatoes in remaining extra-virgin olive oil. Add fresh oregano, salt and black pepper. Place on heavy-duty aluminum foil, seal and grill for about 3 minutes.

Marinade swordfish in citrus-herb vinaigrette. Grill on hot fire for about 5 minutes on one side and 3 minutes on the other, or until done as desired.
Serves 4. One plate of grilled swordfish (250 Calories) with potatoes (100 Calories), cherry tomatoes (45 Calories) and steamed spinach (50 Calories) totals 445 Calories.

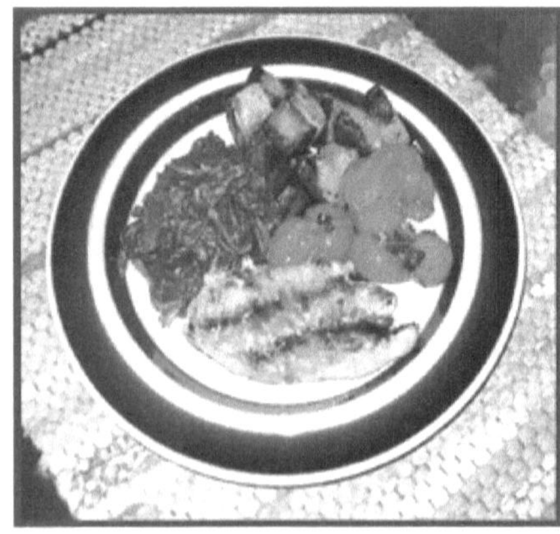

Day 19 - Recipe

Chinese Dinner - Out

No recipe today. No cooking today. Have a Chinese dinner at your favorite restaurant, but make sure you choose a restaurant where you have a reasonable chance to achieve your calorie goal. For today, **your goal for dinner is a maximum of 640 Calories**. This includes any appetizer, soup, main course and any dessert.

Tips for Eating Chinese: You can consume a lot of calories in a Chinese restaurant – if you order carelessly. For example a typical portion of General Tso's chicken is loaded with about 1000 Calories, then add another 200 Calories for a cup of rice.

First rule, order simple. Look for an entree with lots of vegetables, some fish or chicken and brown rice. Tell the waiter you want your food steamed with any sauce on the side. (This is not only a low-calorie way of eating Chinese food but is also the most nutritious way to eat Chinese food.)

Then, knowing your 640 Calorie objective, and that chicken and fish are about 50 Calories per ounce, most steamed vegetable servings average approximately 50 Calories per cup, and rice is about 200 Calories per cup, decide how much of the meal you can eat – and take the remainder home. (Note that you will be eating half a serving of left over Chinese food for lunch tomorrow.) To stay within your maximum allowable calorie total, you should pass on dessert and have the evening snack specified for that day in the diet.

Incidentally, although Chinese is specified, feel free to substitute Thai food, Vietnamese, Indian, Middle Eastern, or any other favorite ethnic food. Just make sure you don't exceed the maximum allowable 640 calories for this meal.

<u>Diet Tip of the Day:</u> Another dilemma for dieters is **judging portion size**. It makes no sense to worry about whether to apportion 70 or 80 Calories per ounce for a cut of lean meat if you have no idea whether the portion you are planning to eat weighs four or ten ounces. To be successful, you must learn to estimate portion sizes with reasonable accuracy.

Day 20 - Recipe

Quick Pasta alla Puttanesca

This famous pasta dish originated in Naples Italy. Puttanesca means "ladies of the night." Although the exact origin of the name is unclear, one thing is clear: It's delicious! Here is one of many recipe versions.

½ pound spaghetti (whole wheat preferred)

20 black or green pitted olives

14.5-oz can diced tomatoes

4 oz tomato sauce

2 tablespoon extra-virgin olive oil

3 cloves of garlic, chopped

1 tablespoon dried minced onion

½ teaspoon crushed red pepper flakes

1 tablespoon capers drained and rinsed

¼ cup currants

Cook spaghetti according to package directions. Drain and return spaghetti to pot; add a teaspoon extra-virgin olive oil and toss to coat.

Heat remaining olive oil in large skillet over medium-high heat. Add red pepper flakes; cook and stir 1 to 2 minutes or until sizzling. Add onion and garlic; cook and stir 1 minute. Add canned tomatoes with juice, tomato sauce, olives, currants and capers. Cook over medium-high heat, stirring frequently, until sauce is heated through.

Serves 4. About 345 Calories per serving

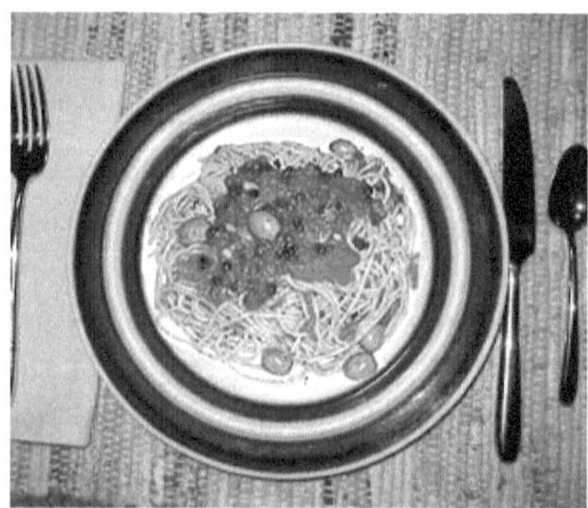

Diet Tip of the Day: Dilute fruit juices, such as apple juice, orange, etc. with water. This cuts the flavor slightly but really reduces calorie content.

Day 21 - Recipe
Frozen-Meat Dinner

No recipe today. No cooking today. Another day off! That's it. At this writing, there are just not that many frozen meat dinners for sale at supermarkets, although new entrees are being introduced continually. Here are some reasonably good frozen-meat dinners:

Steak Portobella	**Lean Cuisine**	**160**
Asian Style Beef & Broccoli	**Smart Ones**	~~**160**~~ **170**
Beef Merlot	**Healthy Choice**	**180**
Homestyle Beef Pot Roast	**Smart Ones**	**180**
Salisbury Steak w Mac & Cheese	**Lean Cuisine**	~~**270**~~ **290**
Pasta with Swedish Meatballs	**Smart Ones**	~~**280**~~ **290**
Classic Meat Loaf	**Healthy Choice**	**300**

If you choose most of the above entrees, you will fall well short of the **300 Calories allocated for this day**. In this case, use the remaining calories anyway you wish. Indulge on extra dessert or save the calories for another day.

See **Appendix B** on page 138 for our comprehensive list of frozen entrees. Please read the important **Frozen-Food Safety Warning** in **Appendix C** on page 143.

<u>**Diet Tip of the Day:**</u> **Understanding nutrition** is not only vital for good health but also will help you control your weight over the long term. For example, did you know that foods that are labeled an "excellent source" of a particular nutrient provide 20% or more of the Recommended Daily Value. Whereas, foods that are a "good source" of a nutrient provide between 10 and 20% of the Recommended Daily Value.

Day 22 - Recipe

<u>Shrimp & Spinach Salad</u>

2 pounds shrimp in shell
½ pound small green beans, trimmed
½ pound baby spinach leaves
2 tablespoon lemon juice
¼ cup extra-virgin olive oil
2 teaspoon minced fresh dill
1 tablespoon minced green onion

To make vinaigrette, combine lemon juice, olive oil, dill, salt and black pepper to taste and whisk until blended. Stir in minced onion and set aside. Steam green beans and set aside.

Peel, de-vein and butterfly shrimp. Place shrimp in a bowl and add water to cover. Add 1 teaspoon of salt, and let stand for 10 minutes. Drain, rinse, drain again, and dry. Arrange shrimp in broiling pan without a rack. Brush shrimp with a little of the vinaigrette and place under preheated broiler, about 3 inches from heat. Broil about 3 to 4 minutes, turning shrimp once, or until both sides turn pink.

Remove shrimp from broiler and add remaining vinaigrette and green beans to the broiling pan. Stir to coat shrimp and beans with vinaigrette. Pour warm vinaigrette over spinach and toss quickly. Plate the spinach and arrange shrimp and green beans on top.
<u>Serves 4</u>. 310 Calories per serving.

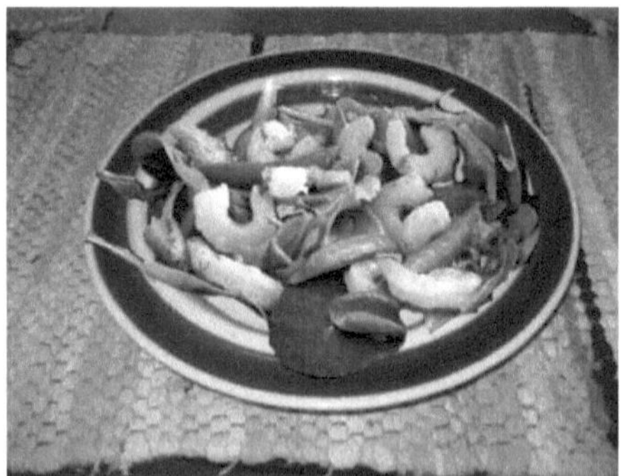

<u>Diet Tip of the Day:</u> After company leaves, have them take some of the leftover food (particularly the dessert) with them – or take the leftovers to work the next day.

<u>Beans & Greens Salad</u>

⅓ cup chopped oregano
⅓ cup chopped parsley
3 cloves garlic, chopped
1 lemon, juiced

Prepare dressing by combining above ingredients and stirring in ¼ cup extra-virgin olive oil. Salt and black pepper to taste.

½ pound mesclun mix
¼ pound green beans
19-oz can garbanzo beans (chickpeas)

Arrange mesclun mix, garbanzo beans and green beans on large platter. Drizzle dressing over beans and greens.
<u>Serves 4</u>. Approximately 260 Calories per serving.

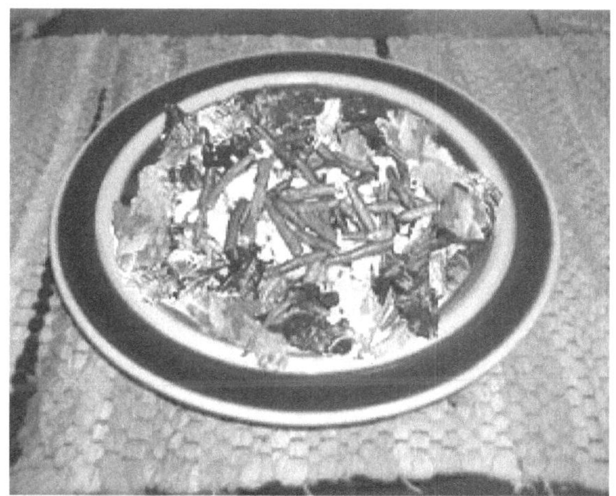

<u>Diet Tip of the Day:</u> Beans are a wonderful food but **beans are an incomplete protein**. If however beans are eaten with a whole-grain bread, the combination forms a complete protein – just as complete and nutritious as meat, poultry, or fish.

Day 24- Recipe

<u>Four-Bean Plus Salad</u> (This is a side dish)

Note that the total caloric value of the salad will change very little, if the proportions of the bean varieties and corn are varied – according to taste.

½ cup canned red kidney beans, drained and rinsed

½ cup canned black beans, drained and rinsed

½ cup canned chick peas, drained and rinsed

½ cup canned cannelloni beans, drained and rinsed

½ cup canned corn, drained

1 small red pepper, chopped

1 small green pepper, chopped

2 tablespoons extra-virgin olive oil

2 tablespoons lemon juice

In a large bowl mix red kidney beans, black beans, chick peas, cannelloni beans, corn and chopped red and green peppers. Stir in olive oil and lemon juice and plate.

<u>Serves about 6</u>. One serving is ½ cup – with about 135 Calories per serving

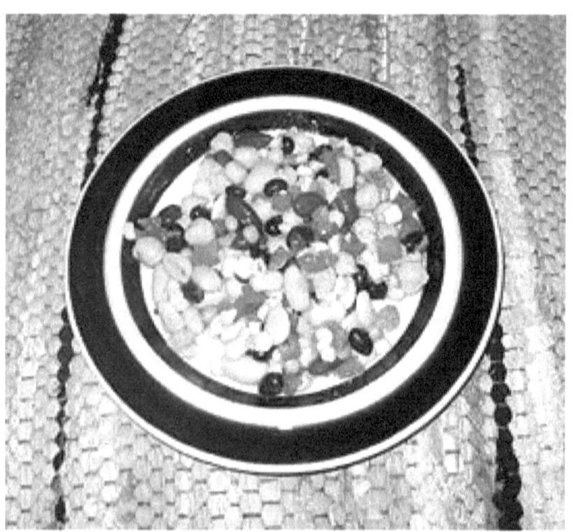

<u>Diet Tip of the Day:</u> Vigorous exercise doesn't necessarily stimulate you to overeat. Just the opposite. In many cases, exercise actually helps curb your appetite – immediately following a workout.

Pan-Broiled Hanger Steak

1¼ pounds hanger steak, well trimmed of fat
¼ cup lime juice
8 small new potatoes, peeled and halved
½ pint cherry tomatoes (about 15), halved

Season both sides of steak with salt and pepper and place in sealable plastic bag with lime juice. Refrigerate for about one hour.

Boil potatoes about 10 minutes. Rinse in cold water. Sauté potatoes in small amount of vegetable oil over medium-high heat until brown.

Sauté cherry tomatoes in small amount of olive oil over medium-high heat until skin begins to crack. Season with chopped fresh basil.

Heat a skillet over medium-high heat. Sear hanger steak on one side for about 5 minutes. Turn over and sear other side approximately 5 minutes (for medium done). Pour off any fat that may have accumulated. Cut into ½-inch slices.

Serves 4. About 320 Calories per serving (for the hanger steak only)

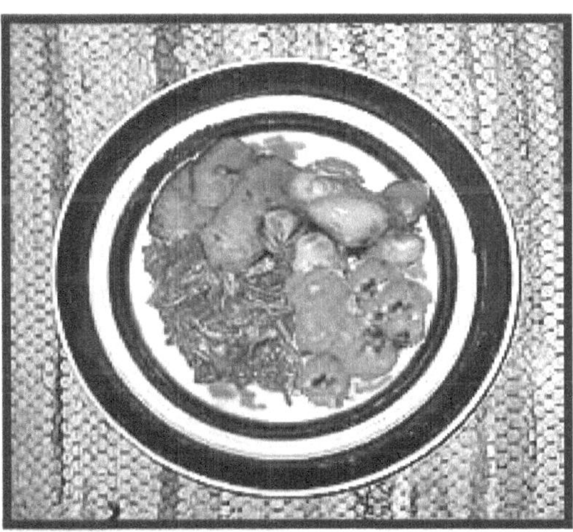

Diet Tip of the Day: If you go to a **party**, don't stand near the food! Be aware of the temptation. Make the effort, and you'll find you eat less.

Day 26 - Recipe

<u>Tina's Grilled Scallops &Polenta</u>

1 pound sea scallops
¾ cup polenta cornmeal
¾ cup skim milk
1 medium portobello mushroom
½ pound green beans
¼ cup chopped red onion
16 asparagus spear
1 teaspoon extra-virgin olive oil
Bring 1½ cups of water and skim milk to rapid boil. Add salt to taste
and slowly add polenta while stirring. Reduce heat. Continue stirring
until desired consistency is reached. Pour polenta into lightly greased
pan. After polenta has cooled cover and refrigerate. Cut chilled
polenta into 4 pieces. Grill on medium-hot fire – about two minutes on
each side.

Brush portobello mushroom and asparagus spear with olive oil and
place on grill for about 3 minutes on each side.

Grill scallops on medium-hot fire. Turn after two minutes or when first
side turns opaque. Grill until second side turns opaque – about another
2 minutes. Don't overcook but test a scallop by cutting to make sure
it's cooked through. Salt and pepper to taste.
<u>Serves 4.</u> The food on the plate pictured below totals about 380
Calories.

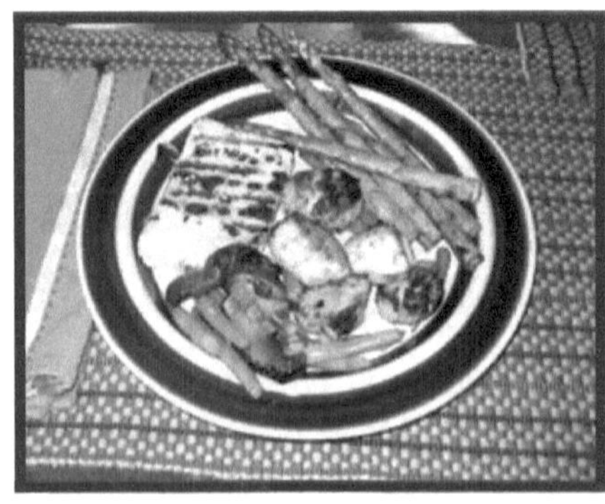

<u>Diet Tip of the Day:</u> To have better control of what you eat **bring your
lunch to work**.

<h1 align="center">Day 27 - Recipe</h1>

<u>Fettuccine in Summer Sauce</u>

This sauce is often served in the summer because it's lighter than what is usually dished up with pasta. But despite its name the sauce is wonderful year round.

½ lb fettuccine
8 oz fresh asparagus, trimmed & cut in 2-inch pieces
¾ pint cherry tomatoes (about 20), halved
2 Tbsp plus 1 tsp extra-virgin olive oil, divided
2 cloves of garlic, chopped
½ small onion, diced

Cook fettuccine according to package directions. Drain and return pasta to pot; add a teaspoon of the olive oil and toss to coat. Meanwhile steam asparagus and drain.

In large skillet over medium-high heat, sauté cherry tomatoes in remaining 2 tablespoons of olive oil until skin begins to crack. Add onion and cook until translucent. Stir in garlic. Thin sauce with pasta liquid to desired consistency. Toss cooked pasta and asparagus into sauce and serve immediately.

<u>Serves 4</u>. About 290 Calories per serving

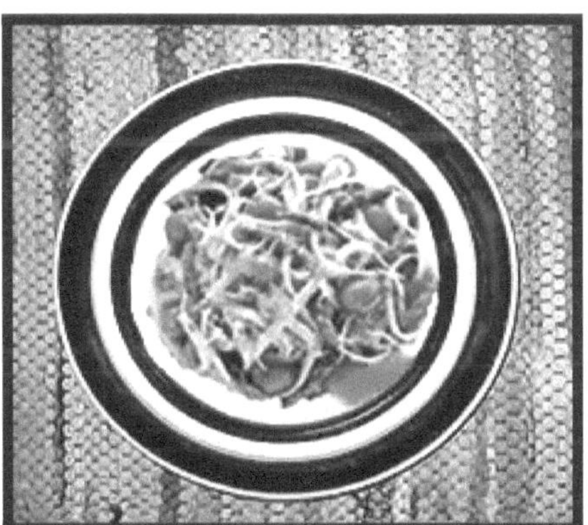

<u>**Diet Tip of the Day:**</u> A major weight-loss fallacy is that you can **get rid of abdominal fat** by working your abdominal muscles. This is based on the incorrect belief that fat is eliminated from a particular part of your body if you engage the muscles underneath that layer of fat. No such luck.

103

Day 28 - Recipe

<u>Frozen Chicken Dinner</u>

No recipe today. No cooking today. Another day off! There are
plenty of frozen chicken choices in your local supermarket. Here are
some reasonably good selections:

Crustless Chicken Pot Pie	**Smart Ones**	~~200~~ 190
Buffalo Style Chicken	**Lean Cuisine**	~~200~~ 190
Home Style Chicken & Potatoes	**Healthy Choice**	200
Honey Balsamic Chicken	**Healthy Choice**	210
Sesame Stir Fry with Chicken	**Lean Cuisine**	280
Roasted Turkey Breast	**Lean Cuisine**	~~280~~ 290
Apple Cranberry Chicken	**Lean Cuisine**	280
Chicken Fettuccini Alfredo	**Healthy Choice**	280
Grilled Chicken Marinara	**Healthy Choice**	280
Sweet & Spicy Orange Chicken	**Healthy Choice**	280
Chicken Parmesan	**Smart Ones**	280
Turkey Breast with Stuffing	**Smart Ones**	280

If you fall short of the **300 Calories allocated for today's frozen
meal**. In this case, use the remaining 100 or so calories anyway you
wish. Splurge on extra dessert or save the calories for another day.

See **Appendix B** on page 138 for our comprehensive list of frozen
entrees. Please read the important **Frozen-Food Safety Warning** in
Appendix C on page 143.

Day 29 - Recipe

<u>Barbequed Shrimp & Corn</u>

   1½ pounds large shrimp, peeled and de-veined

   3 Tbsp of your favorite bottled barbeque sauce

   4 medium ears of corn

Pour barbeque sauce into shallow bowl. Toss shrimp in barbeque sauce to coat. Place shrimp on medium-hot grill. Turn shrimp after about two minutes or when shrimp turn pink. Grill until second side turns pink – approximately another 2 minutes. Don't overcook but test a shrimp by cutting to make sure it is cooked through. Salt and pepper to taste. Serve hot or at room temperature.

<u>**Serves 4**</u>. About 160 Calories per serving (shrimp only).

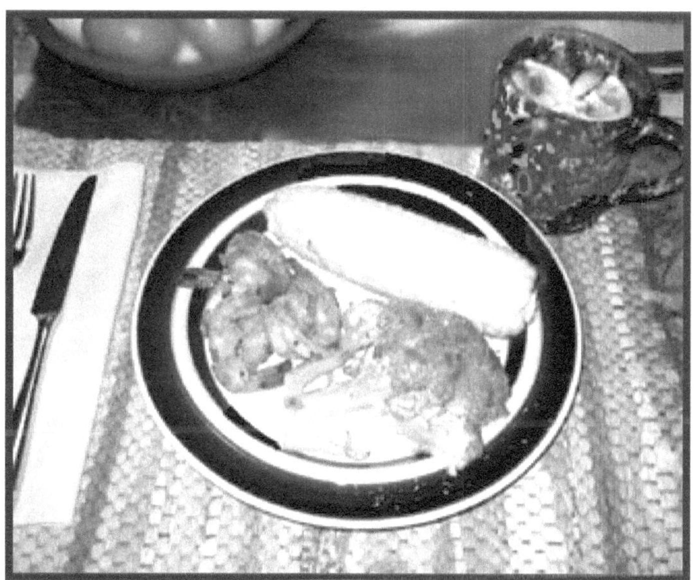

<u>**Diet Tip of the Day:**</u> A very **important weight-profile parameter** is your waist-to-hip ratio. Health risks for heart attack and stroke increase considerably for men with a ratio above 1.0 and for women with a ratio above 0.8. To calculate your ratio, measure your waist size (at its narrowest circumference) and divide it by your hip size (at the widest section).

Day 30 - Recipe

<u>Cheeseburger Heaven</u>

There's really not much to grilling hamburgers. The ideal meat for a juicy burger is ground chuck with about 20% fat, but we are talking diet here. So we opt for leaner, much leaner meat.

1¼ pounds ground sirloin (95% lean)
4 thin slices low-fat American cheese

Mix ground beef in large bowl. Salt and pepper to taste. Divide into 4 equal portions and form burgers about 1-inch thick.

Cook burgers over a hot fire on charcoal or gas-fired grill. For medium, cook about 4 minutes on each side. Top with slice of cheese. Add lettuce and tomato. Season to taste.

<u>Serves 4</u>. About 370 Calories per serving (cheeseburger only).

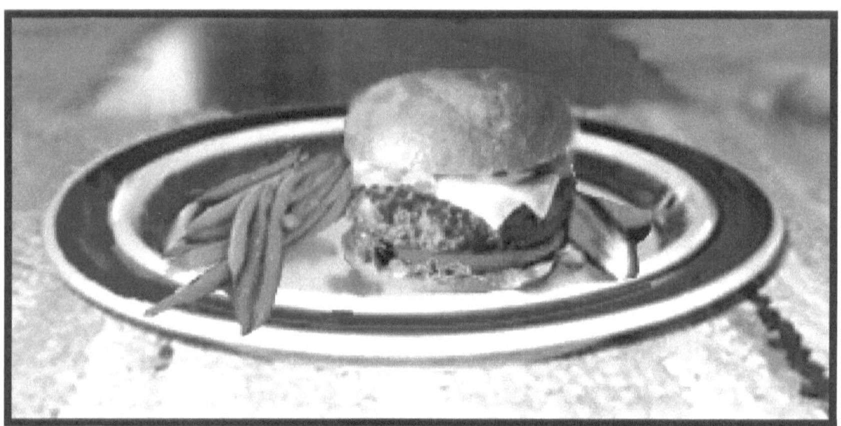

<u>Diet Tip of the Day:</u> **Plan to be on a diet the rest of your life**. Not necessarily a weight-reducing diet. At some point you'll want to just maintain your weight. But you will still need to continue to make good healthy food choices – and not slip back to your old eating habits.

Day 31 - Recipe

Tina's Baked Sea Bass

   4 4-ounce Chilean sea bass fillets
   ½ pound green beans
   ¾ pint cherry tomatoes (about 20)
   ¾ cup brown rice (prepare per package directions)

Sea Bass: Dust filets with flour. Dip in egg wash & then Panko bread crumbs. Place fillets in baking dish coated with non-stick spray. Bake about 15 minutes in oven preheated to 350 °F.

Green Beans & Tomato: Place green beans in skillet. Add ¼-inch of water and cook over medium heat until water boils off. Add cherry tomatoes and olive oil. Stir well and sauté for a few minutes. Season with fresh rosemary and oregano.

Brown Rice-Pesto mix: Prepare brown rice per package directions. Add 4 teaspoons packaged "green" pesto. Mix thoroughly.

Red Pepper Sauce: Blend one roasted red pepper (skinned), ½ cup non-fat yogurt, 1 tsp lemon juice, 1 Tbsp olive oil, 1 Tbsp chili sauce, and a dash of Worcestershire sauce.

Serves 4. One plate consisting of one sea bass fillet with spooned over red pepper sauce (150 Calories), green beans & tomato mix (75 Calories), brown rice-pesto mix (120 Calories) and half ear of corn (50 Calories) – totals about 395 Calories.

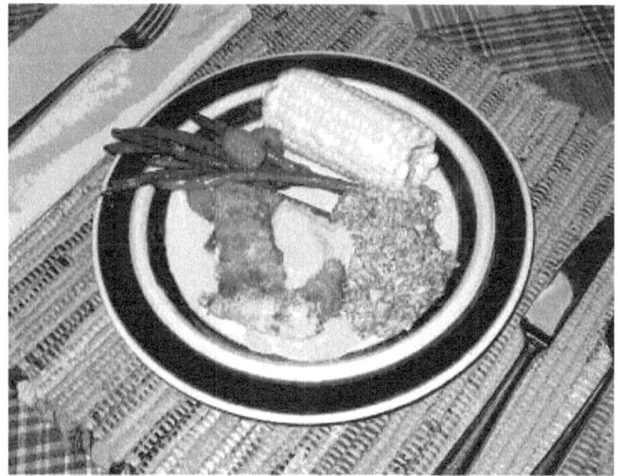

<u>**Diet Tip of the Day:**</u> Protein foods make you **feel full longer** and help prevent overeating.

Day 32 - Recipe

Turkey Tenders & Vegetables

2   turkey breast tenderloins (about 1½ lb)
1   medium eggplant (about ¾ lb)
¾   pound yellow (summer) squash
2   medium plum tomatoes, quartered

<u>Marinade</u>: Whisk in a bowl 2 tsp lemon zest, ¼ cup lemon juice, 2 Tbsp olive oil, 1 Tbsp chopped garlic, 1 Tbsp chopped rosemary, ¼ tsp salt and a pinch of black pepper. Put marinade and turkey breasts in large re-sealable plastic bag. Refrigerate about 45 minutes

Slice eggplant and squash lengthwise about ½-inch thick. Place with tomatoes on a baking sheet coated with a nonstick spray.

Grill turkey breasts approximately 7 to 9 minutes per side, or until an instant-read thermometer inserted from the side to middle registers 160°F. Slice turkey and set aside.

Grill eggplant and zucchini about 4 minutes per side, or until just tender. Grill tomatoes about 2 minutes per side, or until charred but not soft. Cut vegetables bite-size and toss with remaining marinade. Serve with sliced turkey.

<u>Serves 4</u>. About 350 Calories per serving (includes turkey and veggies)

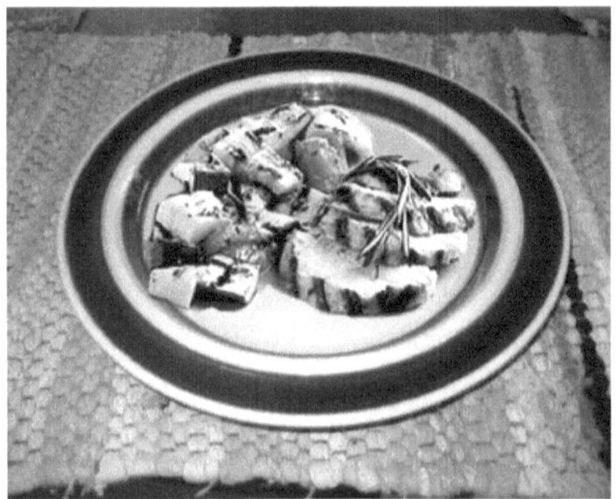

<u>Diet Tip of the Day:</u> It's a lot easier to eat 1000 Calories than it is to burn 1000 Calories exercising. So a stroll after dinner isn't going to offset the calories you ingested eating a Big Mac plus fries.

Day 33 - Recipe

Frozen-Fish Dinner

No recipe today. No cooking today. It's your day off! Some reasonably good frozen fish dinners are:

Shrimp Alfredo	**Lean Cuisine**	230 240
Tuna Noodle Casserole	**Smart Ones**	250 270
Shrimp & Angel Hair Pasta	**Lean Cuisine**	280 290
Parmesan Crusted Fish	**Lean Cuisine**	290 300
Tortilla Crusted Fish	**Lean Cuisine**	300 310

That's it. At this writing, there are just not that many frozen fish dinners for sale at supermarkets, although new entrees are being introduced continually. If you choose any of the above entrees, you will not use all of the **340 Calories allocated for this meal**. In this case, use the excess calories anyway you wish. Splurge on extra dessert or save the calories for another day!

See **Appendix B** on page 198 for our comprehensive list of frozen entrees. Please read the important **Frozen-Food Safety Warning** in **Appendix C** on page 203.

<u>**Diet Tip of the Day:**</u> It's amazing how many people tend to confuse thirst with hunger. This often results in overeating when actually drinking water might be the solution. So, the next time you have a seemingly uncontrollable food craving, try drinking a glass of water instead.

Day 34 - Recipe

<u>Pasta Rapini</u>

2 cloves garlic - coarsely chopped
1½ cups of crushed San Marzano tomatoes
2 cups Rapini (broccoli rabe)
1 tablespoon crushed red pepper flakes (optional)
½ pound medium-sized whole wheat pasta
<u>Tomato Sauce:</u> In large pan, sauté two tablespoons olive oil over medium-high heat. Add the garlic and sauté until translucent (but not browned). Add crushed San Marzano tomatoes (use plum tomatoes if San Marzano are not available) and bring to a boil. Reduce heat to low and simmer for about 30 minutes or until cooked. Season with salt and pepper. Set aside.

<u>Rapini:</u> Discard the tough stems and slice into 2-inch pieces. Bring a pot of water to a boil. Add Rapini (a variety of the vegetable broccoli rabe) and 1 tablespoon salt. Blanch Rapini about 5 minutes or until slightly cooked but still crunchy at stems. Drain, set aside and cover.

Cook pasta according to package instructions until al dente. Three minutes before pasta is ready, add the Rapini to the sauté pan (containing the tomato sauce). Heat mixture over medium heat. Drain pasta and add it to the pan with the Rapini and tomatoes. Add hot pepper flakes (optional) and toss for 1 to 2 minutes over high heat. Drizzle lightly with extra virgin olive oil and plate. Delicious!
Serves 4. About 290 Calories per serving

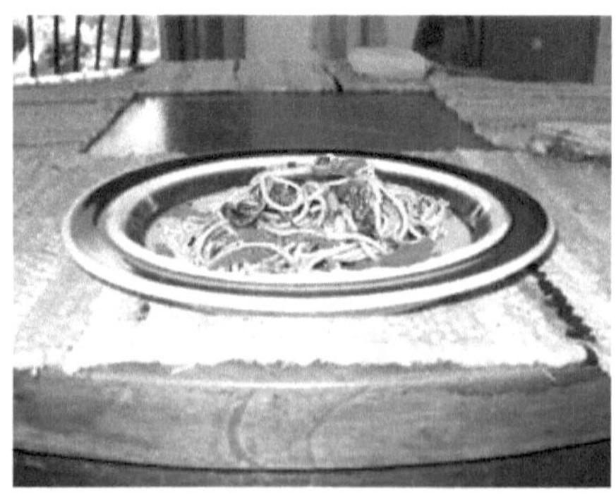

<u>**Diet Tip of the Day:**</u> Keep a daily food log to **record everything you eat**. For some people it really works wonders.

Day 35 - Recipe

Chicken Dinner - Out

No recipe today. No cooking today. Have a chicken dinner at your favorite restaurant, but make sure you choose a restaurant where you have a fighting chance to achieve your calorie goal. For your chicken dinner out, your maximum allowable calories (includes appetizer, soup, main course and dessert) are as follows:
- For the **1200 Calorie Diet**: 530 Calories
- For the **1500 Calorie Diet**: 630 Calories
- For the **1800 Calorie Diet**: 630 Calories

Tips for Eating Chicken Out: First, order simple and order skinless white meat only, such as broiled chicken breast with steamed vegetables and brown rice. (Incidentally, feel free to substitute skinless white meat turkey for chicken.) Tell the waiter you want no sauce, no gravy, nothing added. Then, knowing your calorie objective, and that chicken is about 50 Calories per ounce, most steamed vegetable servings average approximately 50 Calories per cup, and rice is about 100 Calories per ½ cup, decide how much to eat – and take the remainder home. If fresh fruit is not an option, pass on dessert and have the evening snack specified for that day in this diet.

In a restaurant, some nutritionists recommend you eat the low-calorie items on your plate first. Start with the salad, soup and veggies. By the time you get to the chicken and starches you will hopefully be full enough to be content with smaller portions of the higher-calorie choices.

Finally, some dieticians advise their dieting clients not to eat out. That's right. They believe eating at home is safer. But our thought is you have to eat out eventually so why not learn how while your resolve is high?

Diet Tip of the Day: To determine your frame size, circle your wrist with your thumb and third finger. If the tips of your fingers overlap, you have a small frame. If they just touch you are medium, and if they don't touch you have a large frame.

Day 36 - Recipe

<u>Grilled Tilapia</u>

Tilapia is a mild, white fish that inhabits fresh water. This fish has very low levels of mercury because it's fast-growing, short-lived, and mostly eats a vegetarian diet. According to the Monterey Bay Aquarium, choose tilapia farmed in the U.S., in environmentally friendly systems. "Avoid" farmed tilapia from China and Taiwan, where pollution and weak management are a problem.

4 Tilapia filets (about 6 ounces each)

<u>Marinade</u>: ¾ cup olive oil, ½ lemon, juiced, 1 tablespoons oregano, ½ teaspoon black pepper, ¼ cup red wine vinegar, ½ cup finely chopped parsley, 2 cloves garlic, minced and 2 dashes Tabasco (optional).

Combine all ingredients (except filets) in a large re-sealable plastic bag and shake well. Then place fish filets in the marinade for 30 minutes. Remove fillets from marinade and cook on hot grill for approximately 2 to 3 minutes per side.

<u>Serves 4.</u> About 300 Calories per serving (fish only)

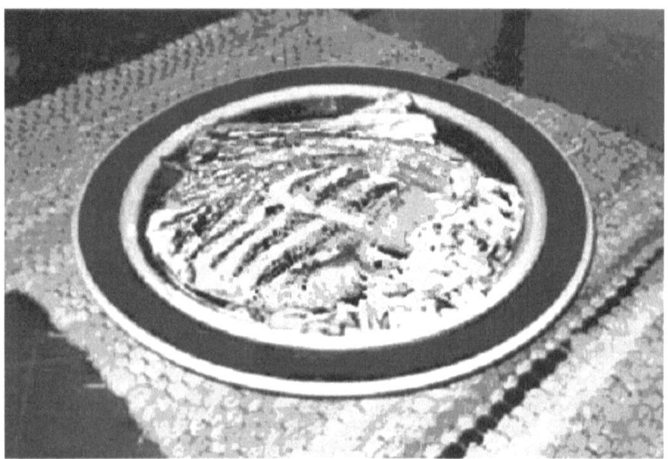

Photo shows two fish filets. Actual serving size is <u>one filet</u>.

<u>Diet Tip of the Day:</u> One serving of asparagus can provide you with 66% of your daily folate needs. Folate is a B-vitamin which is involved with cellular division, and therefore aids the development of a baby's nervous system.

Day 37 - Recipe

Lo-Cal Beef Stew

½ lb beef stew meat, fat trimmed & cut in 1" cubes
2 celery stalks diced
1 medium onion diced
3 large carrots cut into large chunks
3 large boiling potatoes, peeled & cut in chunks
½ up green beans
1 container beef stock (low sodium)
2 tablespoons of flour, and 1 tablespoon of olive oil
½ teaspoon dried herbs, and 1 bay leaf

Season meat with ½ teaspoon dried herbs, salt and pepper. In a Dutch oven, add olive oil and heat until warm. Add meat, diced onion and celery and cook over medium heat about 5 minutes. Add enough beef stock to cover meat. Bring to a boil. Reduce heat, add bay leaf, cover and simmer over low heat until meat is fork tender (about 1½ hours). Add potatoes and carrots. Cover and cook until vegetables are tender (about 30 min). Add green beans and cook an additional 10 min. Skim off any fat from the surface.

In a small bowl, add small amount of water to 2 tablespoons of flour – and stir. Pour the flour-water mixture into the stew and stir until a thick gravy forms. Taste and adjust seasoning. Spoon approximately ¼ of the stew in each plate.

<u>Serves 4</u>. About 365 Calories per serving

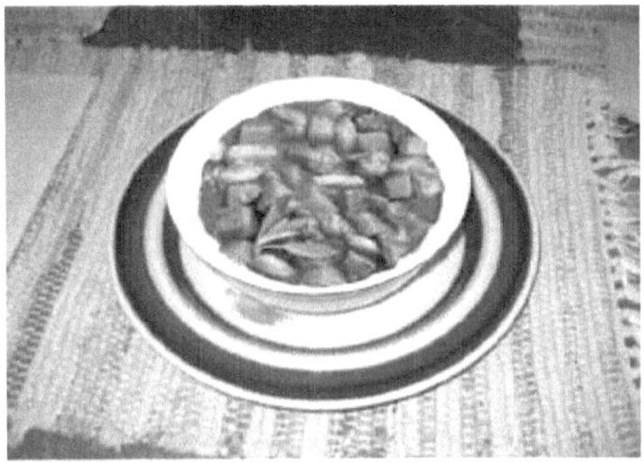

<u>Diet Tip of the Day:</u> **Free-range** animals get more exercise and eat a natural diet, so their meat is usually lower in fat and calories than farm-raised cattle.

<h1 style="text-align:center">Day 38 - Recipe</h1>

Pan-Broiled Lamb Chop

Pan broiling is a quick, easy and a relatively low-calorie technique that can be used to cook many meats.

Start with a rib lamb chop about ¾-inch thick that weighs roughly 6 ounces. Next, it is very important to carefully trim all the visible fat. (After removing the fat and accounting for the bone, about 4 ounces of lean meat should remain.)

Season the chop with salt and ground black pepper. Heat a well-seasoned cast iron or nonstick skillet over high heat. Add the chop (or chops) and cook approximately 4 minutes on each side. (Check center of chop with a small incision to determine when the meat is done.) Plate and serve immediately.

<u>**Serves 1**</u>: About 320 Calories per chop

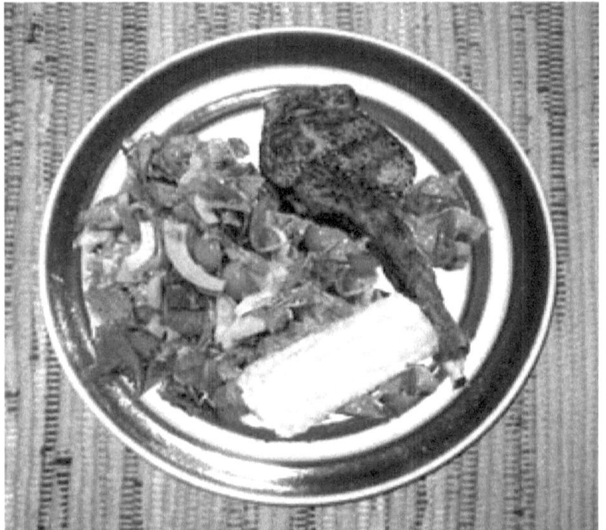

Note corn-on-the-cob is only for the 1800-Calorie diet.

<u>**Diet Tip of the Day:**</u> According to a study published in the Journal of Food Chemistry, broccoli, spinach, kale, Brussels sprouts and other dark green vegetables have the highest cancer-fighting potential found in produce.

<h1 style="text-align:center">Day 39 - Recipe</h1>

<u>Chicken with Veggies</u>

    4 boneless, skinless chicken breast halves (about 5 oz each)
    12 broccoli florets
    1 bunch of asparagus
    2 ripe medium-size tomatoes
    2 tablespoons Lo-Cal (light) salad dressing

Place evenly cut broccoli and asparagus spear in a microwave-safe pan, add a little water to bottom of the pan and top with microwave-safe plastic wrap. (Be sure to pull back one corner of the plastic topper so some steam can escape.) Check veggies periodically and take them out of the microwave when they reach desired softness.

Season chicken breasts evenly with salt and pepper. Heat a large nonstick skillet over medium-high heat. Coat pan with cooking spray. Cook chicken about 4 minutes on each side or until no pink remains.

For each serving, plate one chicken breast and a portion of the steamed broccoli and asparagus. Add one-half of a tomato cut into pieces. Drizzle about 2 tablespoons of a light salad dressing that contains no more than 50 Calories in 2 tablespoons.

<u>Serves 4</u>: One serving of chicken breast halve, veggies & dressing is about 365 Calories.

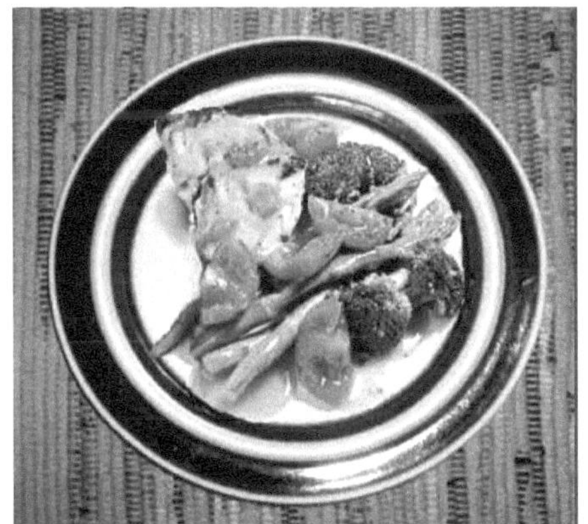

Shown drizzled with Light Thousand Island dressing.

<u>**Diet Tip of the Day:**</u> Steaming in a microwave oven is one of the best ways to cook veggies so they retain nutrients. Another advantage is the cooking adds no fat or sodium.

Day 40 - Recipe

Fish Dinner - Out

No recipe today. No cooking today. Have a fish dinner at your favorite restaurant, but make sure you choose a restaurant where you have a good chance to achieve your calorie goal. For today, your **goal for dinner is a maximum of 595 Calories**. This includes appetizer, soup, main course and dessert.

Tips for Eating Fish Out: The following is almost an exact repeat of the advice given eating out on previous days. First, order simple, such as broiled fish with steamed vegetables and brown rice. Tell the waiter you want no sauce, no gravy, nothing added. Then, knowing your calorie objective, and that fish is about 50 Calories per ounce, most steamed vegetable servings average approximately 50 Calories per cup, and rice is about 100 Calories per ½ cup, decide how much to eat – and take the remainder home. If fresh fruit is not an option, pass on dessert and have the evening snack specified for that day in the diet.

In a restaurant, some nutritionists recommend you eat the low-calorie items on your plate first. Start with the salad, soup and veggies. By the time you get to the fish and starches you will hopefully be full enough to be content with smaller portions of the higher-calorie choices.

Diet Tip of the Day: The average egg has only 210 mg of cholesterol (found in the yoke), contains 80 calories, many vitamins many minerals. If you're healthy and your LDL blood cholesterol level is low, many experts feel you can safely eat one egg per day.

Day 41 - Recipe

Pasta e Fagioli

This is one variation of a traditional, nutritious peasant dish served all over Italy.

    14.5-oz can whole tomatoes with juice, crushed
    14.5-oz can cannellini beans, drained
    1 cup of any tube-shaped pasta
    2 tablespoon olive oil
    1 medium onion, diced
    2 cloves garlic, minced
    1 stalk celery, finely chopped
    3 cups chicken stock
    2 cups fresh baby spinach or escarole
    1 tsp dried basil
    ½ teaspoon dried oregano
    2 Tbsp fresh parsley, chopped

Heat olive oil, onion and celery in large saucepan over medium heat. Sauté until onions are golden brown. Add garlic and stir constantly for one minute. Pour in tomatoes and their juices and bring to a boil. Add beans and chicken stock and return to a boil. Stir in spinach (or escarole) and seasonings. Simmer for about 5 minutes. Add pasta and cook about 15 minutes or until pasta is tender but firm. If needed, thin soup with hot water.

Ladle into soup bowls. Garnish with grated Parmesan cheese. Salt and pepper to taste.

Serves 4. About 300 Calories per serving.

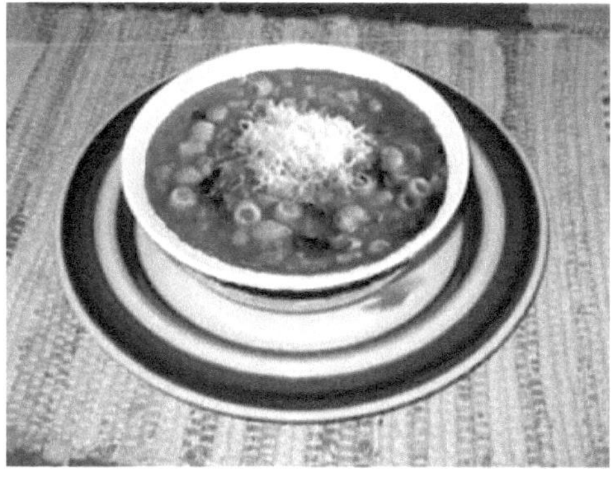

Day 42 - Recipe

Dawn's Blueberry Muffins

Wholesome whole-wheat blueberry muffins just like grandma used to make. Serve them at breakfast, or as a nutritious dessert, or a wonderful snack. (Make a dozen. Have one today and store the remainder in your freezer until they are called for again later in the diet.)

4 ounces bran flakes
¼ cup sugar
1¼ cups whole wheat flour
1 teaspoon baking soda
¼ teaspoon baking powder
¼ teaspoon salt
½ cup blueberries (fresh or frozen)
1 egg, beaten
1 cup buttermilk
¼ cup vegetable oil

Preheat oven to 400 ºF. Coat muffin tins with nonstick cooking spray. In a bowl combine dry ingredients. In another bowl combine wet ingredients and mix thoroughly. Add wet ingredients to dry ingredients and mix until just blended. Do not over mix. Gently fold in blueberries. Spoon batter into muffin tins until two-thirds full. Bake 15 minutes or until muffin tops are golden brown.

Yield is 12 Muffins, 145 Calories each

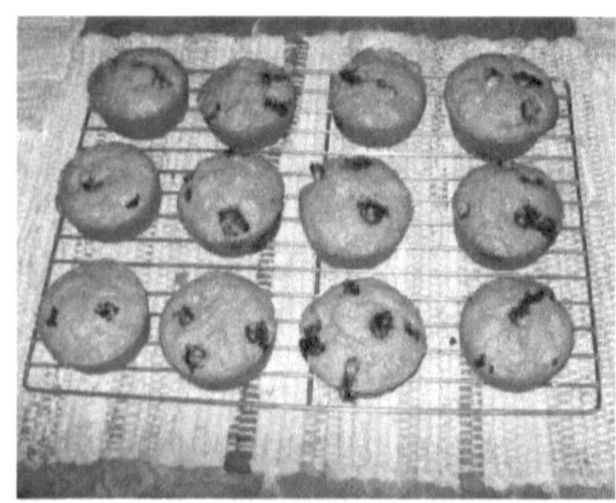

Diet Tip of the Day: **Acquire a good low-calorie cookbook**. Be sure the recipes cover breakfast, lunch and dinner, and all the recipes contain nutritional information, especially the calories per serving.

Day 43 - Recipe

Beef Kebob

- 1 lb boneless beef tenderloin steaks, 1" thick
- 8 ounces medium mushrooms
- 2 medium bell peppers (any color), cut in pieces
- Marinate ingredients:
- 2 tablespoons olive oil
- 1 tablespoon chopped fresh oregano
- 2 cloves garlic, minced
- ½ teaspoon ground black pepper

Cut beef steak into 1-inch square pieces. Combine marinate ingredients in large bowl. Add beef, mushrooms and bell pepper pieces. Toss to coat. Cover bowl and refrigerate for about two hours. Thread beef and vegetable pieces onto eight 12-inch metal skewers.

Grill kebobs over medium-high heat for 8 to 10 minutes, turning occasionally. Check center of meat with a small incision to determine when the meat is done.

Microwave a one-pound package of frozen mixed vegetables. Plate two kebob skewers and about one-quarter of the mixed veggies.
Serves 4. One plate consisting of two kebob skewers (350 Calories) plus ¼ pound of mixed green vegetables (40 Calories) totals about 390 Calories.

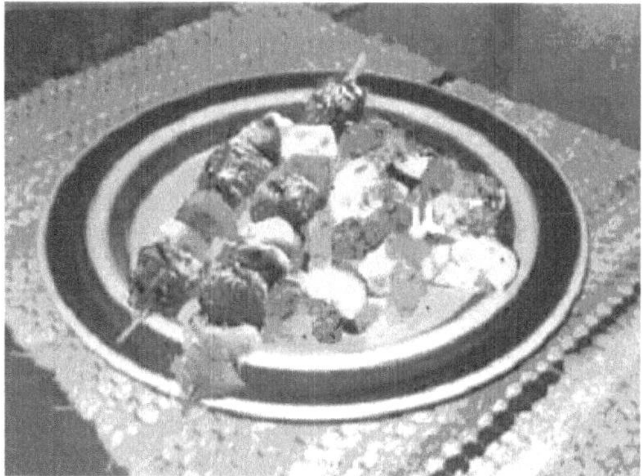

Diet Tip of the Day: Remember your stomach is about the size of your fist. So it doesn't take much food to fill it comfortably.

<u>Baked Haddock</u>

4   4-oz haddock fillets (or salmon fillets)
½ cup white wine
½ cup non-fat yogurt mixed with ¼ cup pureed roasted red pepper
½ pound green beans
¾ pint cherry tomatoes (about 20)
1 tablespoon olive oil
¾ cup bulgur, prepared per package directions

Lightly dust fillets with flour. Dip in beaten egg white and then in Panko bread crumbs. Brown fillets in non-stick pan. Place fillets skin side down in baking dish coated with non-stick spray. Add white wine and cook in oven preheated to 350 °F for about 15 minutes. Spoon pan juices over fillets. Salt and pepper to taste.

Place green beans in skillet. Add ¼-inch of water and cook over medium heat until water boils off. Add cherry tomatoes and olive oil. Stir well and sauté for a few minutes. Season with fresh rosemary and oregano. Salt and pepper to taste.

Plate haddock fillet and spoon over yogurt-red pepper sauce. Garnish with fresh parsley. Add green beans & tomato mix and the bulgur. Serve hot.

<u>Serves 4</u>. One plate consisting of one haddock fillet (215 Calories) with green beans & tomato mix (65 Calories) and bulgur (140 Calories) totals 420 Calories.

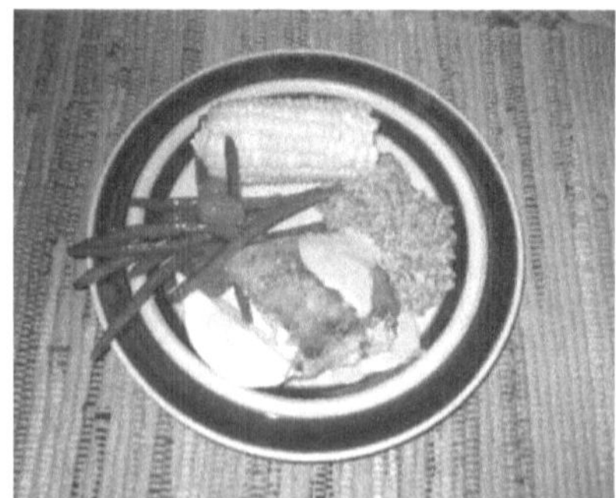

Note that corn-on-the-cob is only for the 1800 Calorie diet.

<u>Diet Tip of the Day:</u> It's much easier to stay with an exercise program when it's done in tandem. So enlist a friend to be your exercise buddy.

Day 45 - Recipe

Chicken Cacciatore

¾ lb skinless, boneless chicken breast halves
¼ lb of your favorite pasta
½ cup chopped onion
½ cup chopped green bell pepper
14.5-ounce can chopped tomatoes, drained
8-ounce can tomato sauce
1½ teaspoons Italian seasoning
⅓ cup sliced ripe olives
⅛ teaspoon black pepper

Cut chicken breasts into small pieces. Spray a large heavy skillet with olive oil flavored cooking spray.

Sauté chicken, onion and green pepper for 6 to 8 minutes. Stir in drained tomatoes and tomato sauce. Add Italian seasoning, olives and ⅛ teaspoon ground black pepper. Mix well to combine. Lower heat and simmer for 15 to 20 minutes, stirring occasionally.

Cook pasta per package directions. Ladle chicken and sauce over pasta and serve immediately.

Serves 4. About 310 Calories per serving

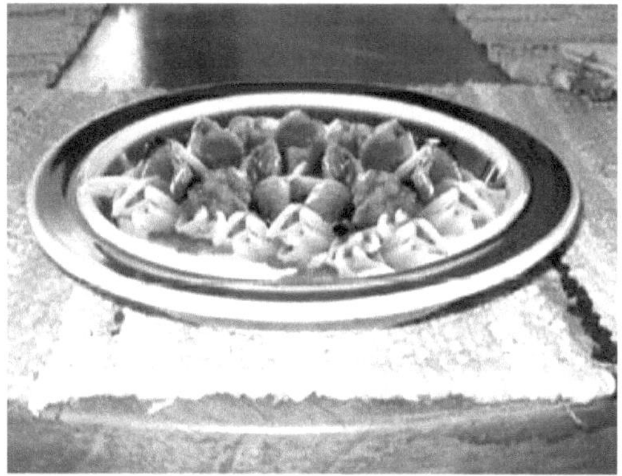

Diet Tip of the Day: Inevitably, you're going to be faced with a stressful situation. Instead of turning to food for comfort, be prepared with some non-food tactics that work for you, such as listening to music, reading, writing in a journal, or meditating.

Day 46 - Recipe
Poached Cod in Tomato Broth

2   cups dry white wine
1   cup clam juice
2   cans (14.5-ounce) diced tomatoes, drained
1   small onion, diced
1   garlic clove, minced
½   tsp dried parsley, or sprigs of fresh parsley
1   bay leaf
12 black olives, pitted and halved
4   cod fish fillets (about 6 ounces each)
Note that sole, flounder, halibut or haddock may be substituted for cod.

Use a pan large enough to hold the fish in a single layer. Place all the ingredients except the fish in the pan. Over high heat, bring poaching liquid to a boil (pan uncovered). Reduce heat and simmer the liquid another 6 minutes.

Carefully place the fish filets in the liquid. Cover the pan and reduce heat until liquid is just simmering. Poach until fish are completely opaque and tender – about 8 minutes. Plate fish and ladle broth over fish.
Serves 4. 275 Calories per serving.

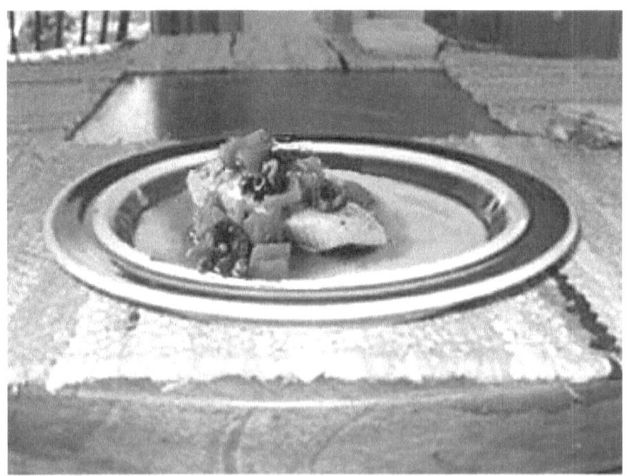

Diet Tip of the Day: A **good reducing diet must help you remain healthy** while you are losing weight.

Day 47 - Recipe

Chinese Dinner - Out

No recipe today. No cooking today. Have a Chinese dinner at your favorite restaurant, but make sure you choose a restaurant where you have a reasonable chance to achieve your calorie goal. For today, **your goal for dinner is a maximum of 640 Calories**. This includes any appetizer, soup, main course and any dessert.

Tips for Eating Chinese: You can consume a lot of calories in a Chinese restaurant – if you order carelessly. For example a typical portion of General Tso's chicken is loaded with about 1,000 Calories, then add another 200 Calories for a cup of rice.

First rule, order simple. Look for an entree with lots of vegetables, some fish or chicken and brown rice. Tell the waiter you want your food steamed with any sauce on the side. (This is not only a low-calorie way of eating Chinese food but is also the most nutritious way to eat Chinese food.)

Then, knowing your 640 Calorie objective, and that chicken and fish are about 50 Calories per ounce, most steamed vegetable servings average approximately 50 Calories per cup, and rice is about 200 Calories per cup, decide how much of the meal you can eat – and take the remainder home. (Note that you will be eating half a serving of left over Chinese food for lunch tomorrow.) To stay within your maximum allowable calorie total, you should pass on dessert and have the evening snack specified for that day in the diet.

Incidentally, although Chinese is specified, feel free to substitute Thai food, Vietnamese, Indian, Middle Eastern, or any other favorite ethnic food. Just make sure you don't exceed the maximum allowable 640 calories for this meal.

Diet Tip of the Day: Inevitably, everyone on a diet hits a frustrating **weight-loss plateau**. Two ways to bust through the plateau are: first to reduce your calorie intake and second to step up your exercise intensity.

Day 48 - Recipe

Healthy Pasta Salad

½ pound fusilli pasta, cooked until tender but firm
2 broccoli crowns, chopped
¼ pint cherry tomatoes (about 8), halved
½ cup black olives, halved
½ cup garbanzo beans (chick peas)
½ cup fresh "light" mozzarella, chopped
1 tablespoon basil
1 tablespoon rosemary
2 teaspoons garlic powder
¼ cup of a **recommended dressing** (page 9)
Combine dry ingredients in a medium-size bowl. Stir in salad dressing.
Mix thoroughly. Salt and black pepper to taste.
<u>Serves 4</u>. 370 Calories per serving.

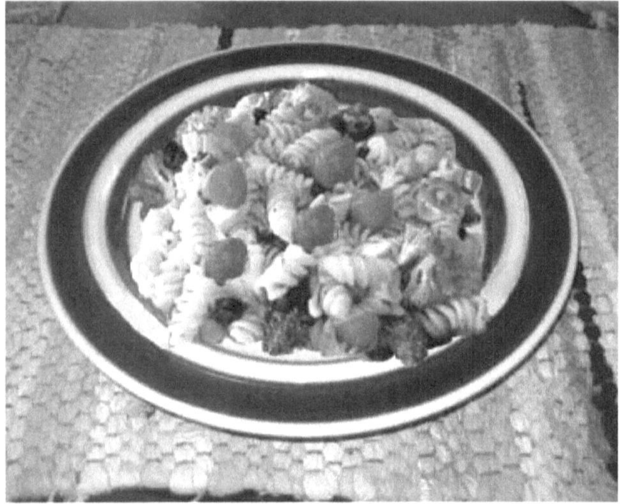

<u>**Diet Tip of the Day:**</u> Ask yourself: "**Why am I overweight**?" Do you eat too much of everything? Too much dessert? Drink too much beer? Is your only exercise walking from the TV to the refrigerator? Determine the why and then focus on one or two of your problem areas. Sometimes it's that simple.

Day 49 - Recipe

Frozen-Meat Dinner

No recipe today. No cooking today. Another day off! That's it. At this writing, there are just not that many frozen meat dinners for sale at supermarkets, although new entrees are being introduced continually. Here are some reasonably good frozen-meat dinners:

Steak Portobella	**Lean Cuisine**	160
Asian Style Beef & Broccoli	**Smart Ones**	~~160~~ 170
Beef Merlot	**Healthy Choice**	180
Homestyle Beef Pot Roast	**Smart Ones**	180
Salisbury Steak w Mac & Cheese	**Lean Cuisine**	~~270~~ 290
Pasta with Swedish Meatballs	**Smart Ones**	~~280~~ 290
Classic Meat Loaf	**Healthy Choice**	300

If you choose any of the above entrees, you will fall short of the **300 Calories allocated for this day**. In this case, use the remaining calories anyway you wish. Indulge on extra dessert or save the calories for another day.

See **Appendix C** on page 198 for a comprehensive list of frozen entrees. Please read the important **Frozen-Food Safety Warning** in **Appendix C** on page 203.

<u>**Diet Tip of the Day:**</u> Experts agree that whether you are trying to lose weight or just maintain your weight, **it's calories that count**. It doesn't matter what foods the calories are from. To lose weight you must eat fewer calories than you burn. Calories count! Not carbs, not Weight Watchers points. Calories – period!

125

Day 50 - Recipe

Pan-Fried Sole

4   sole fillets (6-ounces each), skinned
1   tablespoon olive oil

Salsa Ingredients:

1 pint cherry tomatoes, quartered
¾ cup cucumber, finely chopped
⅓ cup yellow bell pepper, finely chopped
3 tablespoons fresh basil, chopped
2 tablespoons capers
1½ tablespoons shallots, finely chopped
1 tablespoon balsamic vinegar
2 teaspoons lemon rind, grated

Combine salsa ingredients in a bowl and stir in ½ teaspoon salt and ⅛ teaspoon black pepper. Mix thoroughly.

Heat olive oil in a large nonstick skillet over medium-high heat. Season sole fillets with ½ teaspoon salt and ⅛ teaspoon black pepper. Add fish to pan; cook about 1½ minutes on each side or until fish flakes easily when tested with a fork. Spoon salsa over fish and serve immediately.

Serves 4. 325 Calories per serving

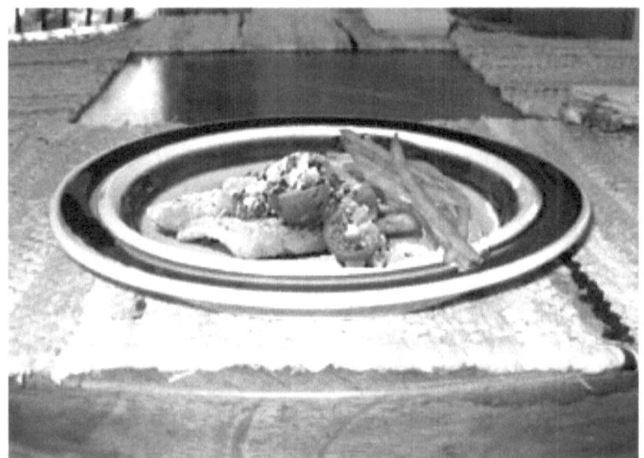

Diet Tip of the Day: If you are overweight start on a weight loss diet now because it will only become **more difficult to lose weight as you get older**.

Day 51 - Recipe

Beans & Greens Salad (Repeated)

⅓ cup chopped oregano
⅓ cup chopped parsley
3 cloves garlic, chopped
1 lemon, juiced

Prepare dressing by combining above ingredients and stirring in ¼ cup extra-virgin olive oil. Salt and pepper to taste.

½ pound mesclun mix
¼ pound green beans
19-ounce can garbanzo beans (chickpeas)

Arrange mesclun mix, garbanzo beans and green beans on a large platter. Drizzle dressing over beans and greens.

Serves 4. Approximately 260 Calories per serving.

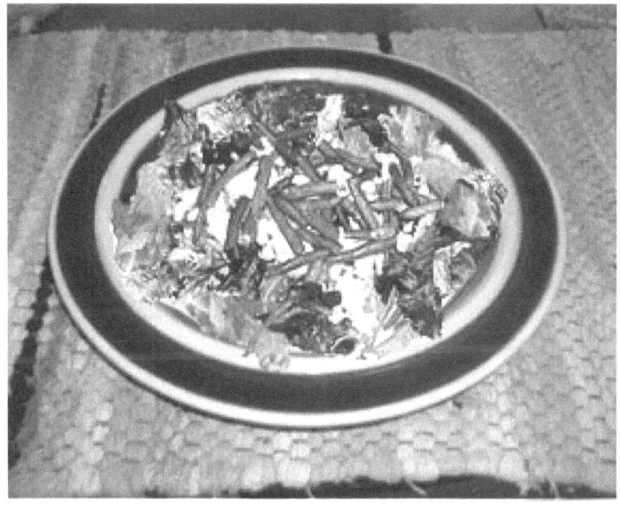

Diet Tip of the Day: Fat-free isn't always your best bet. Low fat doesn't necessarily mean low calorie! Most often sugar is substituted for fat and the calorie total remains the same or even higher. Instead, look for low-calorie or reduced-calorie foods.

Day 52 - Recipe

Chicken Piccata

1 pound boneless skinless chicken breast halves
2 teaspoons olive oil
1 teaspoon minced garlic
¼ cup shallots, diced
¾ pound fresh green beans, washed and snipped
1 teaspoon lemon juice
¼ cup capers, rinsed
2 fresh lemons, cut into small wedges

In a skillet, heat olive oil and minced garlic over medium heat. Sauté chicken breasts and shallots for two to three minutes, tossing often, until chicken is partially cooked. Add green beans and one teaspoon of lemon juice and sauté for an additional two to three minutes, or until chicken is completely cooked and green beans are al dente. Add capers; and cover chicken. Let sit for one more minute to warm capers. Serve immediately with wedges of lemon.

Serves 4. 270 calories per serving

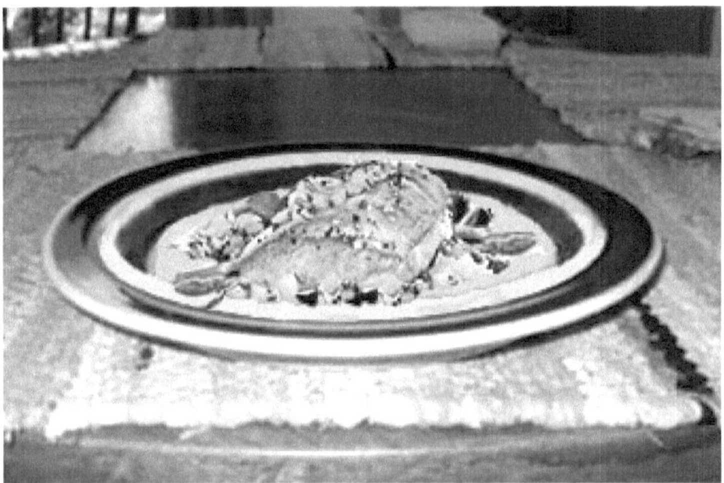

Diet Tip of the Day: Handle **occasional overeating by compensating**. To do this, estimate how far you have strayed from your weight-loss diet and then make amends at the next opportunity (usually the next meal or two) – by eating less.

Day 53 - Recipe

Beef Steak Strips

1 lb top loin sirloin, or top round about ¾" thick
1 tsp garlic, finely chopped
½ tsp dry thyme
½ tsp salt and ¼ tsp black peppercorns

Cut the steak into 3-inch long by ¼-inch thick strips Sprinkle the beef strips with garlic, thyme, salt and pepper. Prepare a large non-stick skillet over medium-high heat. Add the steak strips and shake the skillet constantly to avoid sticking. Cook approximately 2 to 3 minutes until meat is seared but pink inside. Check the center by making small incision.

Serves 4. About 330 Calories per serving (meat only).

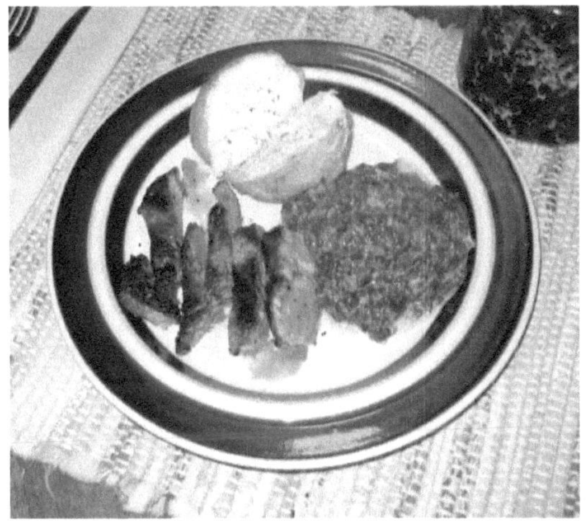

Diet Tip of the Day: Bear in mind, that knowledge and the discipline to **workout regularly** are far more important than fancy equipment.

Day 54 - Recipe
Tina's Grilled Scallops & Polenta

1 pound sea scallops
¾ cup polenta cornmeal
¾ cup skim milk
1 medium Portobello mushroom
½ pound green beans
¼ cup chopped red onion
16 asparagus spear
1 teaspoon extra-virgin olive oil

Bring 1½ cups of water and skim milk to rapid boil. Add salt to taste and slowly add polenta while stirring. Reduce heat. Continue stirring until desired consistency is reached. Pour polenta into lightly greased pan. After polenta has cooled cover and refrigerate. Cut chilled polenta into 4 pieces. Grill on medium-hot fire – about two minutes on each side.

Brush Portobello mushroom and asparagus spear with olive oil and place on grill for about 3 minutes on each side.

Grill scallops on medium-hot fire. Turn after two minutes or when first side turns opaque. Grill until second side turns opaque – about another 2 minutes. Don't overcook but test a scallop by cutting to make sure it's cooked through. Salt and pepper to taste.
Serves 4. The food on the plate pictured below totals about 380 Calories.

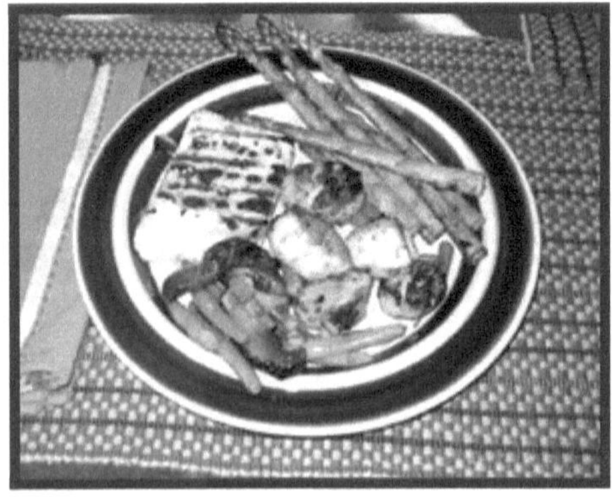

Day 55 - Recipe

<u>Hearty Vegetable Soup</u>

2 15-oz cans white kidney beans, drained
1 tablespoon olive oil
½ large yellow onion, chopped
2 garlic cloves, minced
1 cup chopped fresh tomatoes
2 celery stalks, cut into ½-inch pieces
1½ carrots, cut into ½-inch pieces
5 cups vegetable stock
1 medium potato, cut into ½-inch pieces
¼ cup chopped fresh basil
¼ head of red cabbage, cut into ½-inch pieces
2 zucchini or summer squash, cut into ½-inch pieces

Heat olive oil in a large pot over medium heat. Add onion and garlic.
Sauté 5 minutes. Add green cabbage, tomatoes, celery, and carrots.
Sauté 10 minutes. Add beans, 5 cups of stock, potatoes, and basil.
Bring to a boil. Reduce heat, cover and simmer for one hour. Add red
cabbage, zucchini and salt . Cover and simmer until vegetables are
tender, about 20 minutes longer. Stir in about ¼ cup Parmesan cheese
and sprinkle a dash of Tabasco hot sauce if you want a little zip
<u>Serves 4</u>. 360 Calories per serving

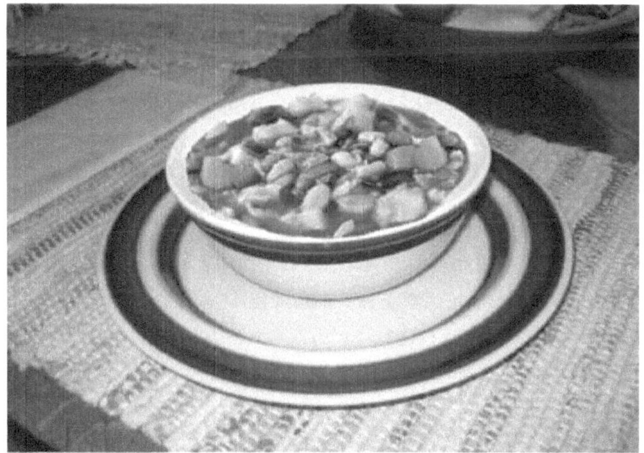

<u>Diet Tip of the Day:</u> Water and fiber contain no calories – that is **zero
Calories** per ounce.

Day 56 - Recipe

<u>Frozen Chicken Dinner</u>

No recipe today. No cooking today. Another day off! There are plenty of frozen chicken choices in your local supermarket. Here are some reasonably good selections:

Crustless Chicken Pot Pie	**Smart Ones**	~~200~~ 190
Buffalo Style Chicken	**Lean Cuisine**	~~200~~ 190
Home Style Chicken & Potatoes	**Healthy Choice**	**200**
Honey Balsamic Chicken	**Healthy Choice**	**210**
Sesame Stir Fry with Chicken	**Lean Cuisine**	**280**
Roasted Turkey Breast	**Lean Cuisine**	~~280~~ 290
Apple Cranberry Chicken	**Lean Cuisine**	**280**
Chicken Fettuccini Alfredo	**Healthy Choice**	**280**
Grilled Chicken Marinara	**Healthy Choice**	**280**
Sweet & Spicy Orange Chicken	**Healthy Choice**	**280**
Chicken Parmesan	**Smart Ones**	**280**
Turkey Breast with Stuffing	**Smart Ones**	**280**

If you choose the first four meals of the above, you will fall far short of the **300 Calories allocated for today's frozen meal**. In this case, use the remaining 100 or so calories anyway you wish. Splurge on extra dessert or save the calories for another day.

See **Appendix C** on page 198 for our comprehensive list of frozen entrees. Please read the important **Frozen-Food Safety Warning** in **Appendix C** on page 203.

Day 57 - Recipe

Salmon with Mango Salsa

    4   salmon fillets (about 5 ounces each)
    1½ pounds baby new potatoes, halved
    1   mango, ripe
    3   green onions, finely chopped
    3   tablespoons chopped fresh cilantro
    2   tablespoons lemon juice
    2   teaspoons extra-virgin olive oil
    4   cups watercress

Remove any tiny bones from salmon. Press crushed peppercorns into flesh side of salmon. Set aside. Place halved potatoes into saucepan. Cover with water and bring to a boil. Reduce the heat and simmer until tender, about 10-12 minutes and drain.

Prepare salsa: Peel and seed the mango. Dice the mango flesh and put into a large bowl. Mix in green onions, cilantro, lemon juice, olive oil, and an optional dash of Tabasco.

Heat a grill pan coated with nonstick cooking spray over medium-high heat. Place salmon fillets in pan, skin-side down. Cook for 4 minutes. Turn fish over and cook until done, about another 4 minutes. Arrange watercress and new potatoes on serving plates. Place salmon on top and spoon over mango salsa.

Serves 4. 460 Calories per serving

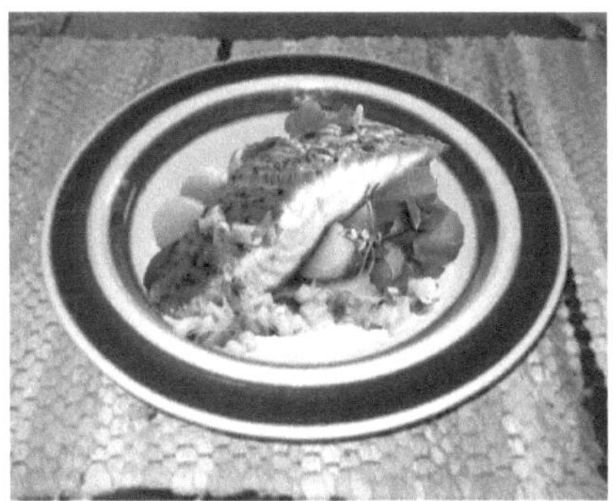

Diet Tip of the Day: All **foods are a combination of water, carbohydrate, protein, fat and fiber**. Knowing this can lead to a better understanding of why a food has a particular caloric value.

Day 58 - Recipe

<u>Pork Chop with Orange Slices</u>

4   loin pork chops, ½-inch-thick (about 1½ lbs total, including bones)
8   orange slices, ¼-inch-thick
1   teaspoon salt
¾   teaspoon black pepper
¼   cup orange marmalade preserve
½   cup bottled fruit-based barbecue sauce
such as Grandville's Gourmet BBQ Sauce
<u>Marinade</u>: ½ cup orange juice, 2 teaspoons soy sauce and ¼ teaspoon crushed red pepper.

Combine pork chops and marinade in large re-sealable plastic bag. Refrigerate for about 30 minutes. Remove chops from marinade and season with salt and black pepper.

Stir together orange marmalade and BBQ sauce in a small bowl. Brush one side of pork chops evenly with half of marmalade-BBQ mixture. Grill chops, with marmalade-BBQ mixture side up over medium-high heat (about 375°) for about 5 minutes or until done. Turn chops, and brush with remaining marmalade-BBQ mixture. Grill another 5 minutes or until done. Grill orange slices over medium-high heat, 1 minute on each side.
<u>Serves 4</u>. 470 Calories per serving (includes pork chop and orange slices).

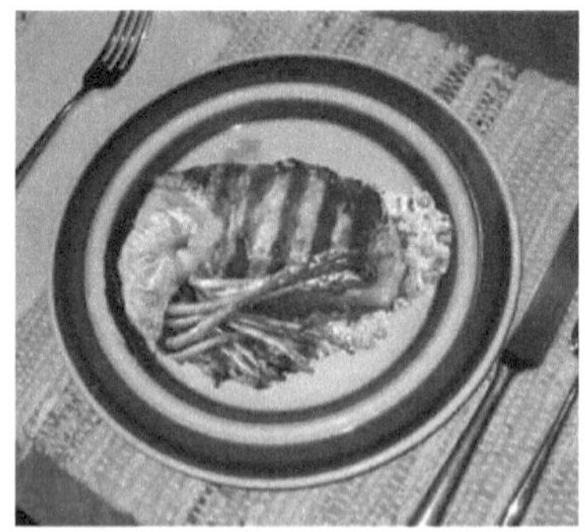

<u>Diet Tip of the Day:</u> Make sure fat is trimmed from meat. Most meats are about 80 Calories per ounce – whereas, pure fat is 256 Calories per ounce!

Day 59 - Recipe

Fish Dinner - Out

No recipe today. No cooking today. Have a fish dinner at your favorite restaurant, but make sure you choose a restaurant where you have a good chance to achieve your calorie goal. For today, your **goal for dinner is a maximum of 595 Calories**. This includes appetizer, soup, main course and dessert.

Tips for Eating Fish Out: The following is almost an exact repeat of the advice given eating out on previous days. First order simple, such as broiled fish with steamed vegetables and brown rice. Tell the waiter you want no sauce, no gravy, nothing added. Then, knowing your calorie objective, and that fish is about 50 Calories per ounce, most steamed vegetable servings average approximately 50 Calories per cup, and rice is about 100 Calories per ½ cup, decide how much to eat – and take the remainder home. If fresh fruit is not an option, pass on dessert and have the evening snack specified for that day in the diet.

In a restaurant, some nutritionists recommend you eat the low-calorie items on your plate first. Start with the salad, soup and veggies. By the time you get to the fish and starches you will hopefully be full enough to be content with smaller portions of the higher-calorie choices.

Diet Tip of the Day: A handful of studies suggest that chewing gum may help reduce your craving for sweet snacks, and cut your caloric intake by about 50 per day. Another study actually showed that gum chewers experienced a small increase in their daily energy expenditure. And gum adds hardly any calories to your diet. Regular gum has about 10 calories and sugar-free varieties about five calories per stick.

Day 60 - Recipe

<u>Chicken Stew over Rice</u>

4   boneless skinless chicken breasts (about 1 lb)
1   medium Onion
3   stalks celery
12 mushrooms
2   cups baby carrots
3   cups broccoli florets
½ teaspoon black pepper
¼ teaspoon herb seasoning blend
2   teaspoons Worcestershire Sauce
1   bay leaf
1   cup Campbell's Cream of Chicken Soup

Prepare a large, heavy, stove-top pot with cooking spray. Sauté at medium-high heat finely chop onion until caramelized. Cut chicken into bite size pieces and add to pot. Cook and toss until chicken is no longer pink. Add black pepper, herb seasoning and Worcestershire sauce. Stir. Add sliced celery and mushrooms, and then broccoli, carrots and bay leaf. Pour in Cream of Chicken soup. Gradually add one cup water while stirring. (You may want to add more water to get consistency desired.) Simmer until hot and flavors have combined. Serve over rice.

<u>Serves 4.</u> 360 Calories per serving (not including the brown rice below the stew).

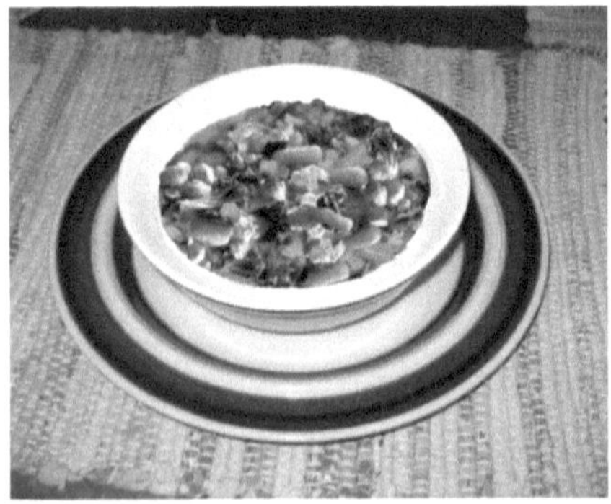

<u>Diet Tip of the Day:</u> Studies show people who eat 5 to 6 **mini-meals** and snacks a day don't feel as hungry and are better able to control their appetite and their weight.

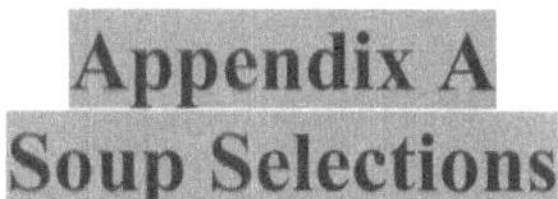

Appendix A
Soup Selections

When the Daily Meal Plan menu specifies soup have only one serving (8 ounces) unless stated otherwise. Note that the listed soups were available in most supermarkets as of 07/21/2020.   *These are a canned soup selections.

Soup Description	Calories
Healthy Choice Chicken with Rice	90
Campbell's Tomato	100
Healthy Choice Country Vegetable	100
Progresso Minestrone*	110
Progresso Chickarina*	110
Progresso Italian-Style Wedding*	120
Campbell's Home-Style Lite Chicken Corn Chowder*	120
Campbell's Home-Style Chicken Noodle	130
Campbell's Home-Style Butter Nut Squash*	130
Campbell's Healthy Request Vegetable Beef	140
Progresso Lentil*	140
Progresso Green Split Pea*	150
Campbell's Slow Kettle New England Clam Chowder	160
Progresso Macaroni and Bean*	160
Progresso New England Clam Chowder*	170
Progresso Lasagna-Style*	170
Progresso Broccoli Cheese with Bacon*	180
Have 2 servings of 90 Calorie soup	180
Campbell's Chunky Classic Chicken Noodle	190
Amy's Rustic Italian Vegetable*	190
Campbell's Chunky Beef n Cheese*	200
Amy's French Country Vegetable*	210
Campbell's Chunky Sirloin Burger + Vegetables	220
Enjoy two servings of a 110 or 120 Calorie soup	230
Enjoy two servings of a 120 Calorie soup	240

Appendix B
Frozen Entrees

Appendix D lists three popular brands of frozen entrées: Healthy Choice, Lean Cuisine and Smart Ones. Note that each brand is color coded. The listing is further divided by entrée type: Poultry entrées, Meat entrées, Seafood entrées, Pasta entrées, Pizza and Other entrées. The entire table is arranged from the lowest to highest in calories. Note that the listed frozen entrées were available as of 08/14/2020.

Type	Name	Brand	Calorie
Poultry	Tomato Basil Chicken & Spinach	Smart Ones	160
Meat	Steak Portobella	Lean Cuisine	160
Meat	Asian Style Beef & Broccoli	Smart Ones	170
Poultry	Herb Roasted Chicken	Lean Cuisine	170
Poultry	Slow Roasted Turkey Breast	Smart Ones	170
Poultry	Creamy Basil Chicken w Broccoli	Smart Ones	170
Poultry	Grilled Chicken Marsala	Healthy Choice	180
Poultry	Garlic Chicken Rolls	Lean Cuisine	180
Meat	Beef Merlot	Healthy Choice	180
Meat	Homestyle Beef Pot Roast	Smart Ones	180
Poultry	Roasted Turkey & Vegetables	Lean Cuisine	190
Poultry	Chicken & Broccoli Alfredo	Healthy Choice	190
Poultry	Chicken & Vegetable Stir Fry	Healthy Choice	190
Other	Broccoli & Cheddar Roast Potato	Smart Ones	190
Poultry	Crustless Chicken Pot Pie	Smart Ones	190
Poultry	Buffalo Style Chicken	Lean Cuisine	190
Poultry	Home Style Chicken & Potatoes	Healthy Choice	200
Pasta	Angel Hair Marinara	Smart Ones	200
Poultry	Salisbury Steak	Smart Ones	200
Meat	Roast Beef & Mashed Potatoes	Smart Ones	200
Pasta	Primavera Pasta	Smart Ones	210

Category	Item	Brand	Calories
Pasta	Ravioli Florentine	Smart Ones	210
Poultry	Cajun Style Chicken & Shrimp	Healthy Choice	220
Pasta	Cheese Ravioli Mushroom Sauce	Smart Ones	230
Poultry	Ranchero Chicken Wrap	Smart Ones	230
Poultry	Lemon Herb Chicken Picante	Smart Ones	230
Pasta	Cheese Ravioli Mushroom Sauce	Smart Ones	230
Meat	Meat Loaf with Mashed Potatoes	Lean Cuisine	240
Seafood	Shrimp Alfredo	Lean Cuisine	240
Poultry	Chicken Margherita	Smart Ones	240
Poultry	Grilled Chicken Caesar	Lean Cuisine	240
Poultry	Honey Glazed Turkey & Potatoes	Healthy Choice	240
Pasta	Spicy Penne Arrabiata	Lean Cuisine	240
Pasta	Four Cheese Cannelloni	Lean Cuisine	250
Poultry	Creamy Basil Chicken w Tortellini	Lean Cuisine	250
Pasta	Cheese Ravioli	Lean Cuisine	250
Pasta	Vermont Cheddar Mac & Cheese	Lean Cuisine	250
Pasta	Fettuccini Alfredo	Smart Ones	250
Poultry	Oriental Chicken	Smart Ones	250
Poultry	Fiesta Grilled Chicken	Lean Cuisine	250
Pasta	Chicken Linguini Red Pepper	Healthy Choice	250
Poultry	Golden Roasted Turkey Breast	Healthy Choice	250
Poultry	Chicken Mesquite	Smart Ones	250
Poultry	Chicken Oriental	Smart Ones	250
Poultry	Orange Sesame Chicken	Smart Ones	250
Poultry	Baked Chicken	Lean Cuisine	260
Poultry	Teriyaki Chicken & Vegetables	Smart Ones	260
Seafood	Tuna Noodle Casserole	Smart Ones	260
Pasta	Spaghetti with Meatballs	Lean Cuisine	260
Poultry	Creamy Chicken & Noodles	Healthy Choice	260
Meat	Barbecue Steak w Red Potatoes	Healthy Choice	260

Pasta	Creamy Rigatoni with Chicken	Smart Ones	260
Pasta	Macaroni & Cheese	Smart Ones	260
Pasta	Butternut Squash Ravioli	Lean Cuisine	260
Other	Santa Fe Rice & Beans	Smart Ones	260
Other	Coconut Chickpea Curry	Lean Cuisine	260
Poultry	Glazed Turkey Tenderloins	Lean Cuisine	270
Poultry	Kung Pao Chicken	Healthy Choice	270
Poultry	Chicken Margherita w Balsamic	Healthy Choice	270
Poultry	Chicken Strips & Sweet Potatoes	Smart Ones	270
Pasta	Sesame Noodles with Vegetables	Smart Ones	280
Pasta	Spaghetti with Meat Sauce	Smart Ones	280
Meat	Salisbury Steak w Mac & Cheese	Lean Cuisine	290
Pasta	Penne Rosa	Lean Cuisine	270
Poultry	Turkey Breast & Stuffing	Smart Ones	280
Pasta	Classic Macaroni & Beef	Lean Cuisine	270
Pasta	Mushroom Mezzaluna Ravioli	Lean Cuisine	270
Other	Asian Pot Stickers	Lean Cuisine	280
Poultry	Sesame Stir Fry w Chicken	Lean Cuisine	280
Poultry	Apple Cranberry Chicken	Lean Cuisine	280
Poultry	Chicken Fettuccini Alfredo	Healthy Choice	280
Poultry	Grilled Chicken Marinara	Healthy Choice	280
Poultry	Sweet & Spicy Orange Chicken	Healthy Choice	280
Poultry	Chicken Parmesan	Smart Ones	280
Poultry	Turkey Breast w Stuffing	Smart Ones	280
Meat	Beef & Broccoli	Healthy Choice	280
Meat	Meatball Marinara	Healthy Choice	280
Meat	Beef Teriyaki	Healthy Choice	280
Pasta	Spinach Artichoke Ravioli	Lean Cuisine	280
Other	Vegetable Fried Rice	Smart Ones	280
Pasta	Spinach Artichoke Ravioli	Lean Cuisine	280

Pasta	Linguini with Ricotta & Spinach	Lean Cuisine	280
Poultry	Chicken Fettuccini	Lean Cuisine	280
Pasta	Spaghetti & Meatballs	Healthy Choice	280
Pasta	Spaghetti with Meat Sauce	Smart Ones	280
Other	Vegetable Fried Rice	Smart Ones	280
Other	Asian Pot Stickers	Lean Cuisine	280
Poultry	Chicken with Almonds	Lean Cuisine	290
Poultry	Chicken w Peanut Sauce	Lean Cuisine	290
Seafood	Shrimp & Angel Hair Pasta	Lean Cuisine	290
Poultry	Grilled Chicken Pesto w Veggies	Healthy Choice	290
Pasta	Pasta w Swedish Meatballs	Smart Ones	290
Poultry	Roasted Turkey Breast	Lean Cuisine	290
Poultry	General Tso's Spicy Chicken	Healthy Choice	290
Poultry	Pineapple Chicken	Healthy Choice	290
Poultry	Chicken Enchiladas Suiza	Smart Ones	290
Meat	Swedish Meatballs	Lean Cuisine	290
Seafood	Lemon Pepper Fish	Healthy Choice	290
Other	Santa Fe Rice & Beans	Smart Ones	290
Pizza	Thin Crust Cheese Pizza	Smart Ones	290
Seafood	Parmesan Crusted Fish	Lean Cuisine	300
Pasta	Santa Fe-Style Rice & Beans	Lean Cuisine	300
Poultry	Roasted Turkey & Vegetables	Lean Cuisine	300
Poultry	Sweet & Sour Chicken	Lean Cuisine	300
Poultry	Crustless Chicken Pot Pie	Healthy Choice	300
Poultry	Sweet Sesame Chicken	Healthy Choice	300
Poultry	Chicken Fettuccini	Smart Ones	300
Poultry	General Tso's Chicken	Smart Ones	300
Meat	Classic Meat Loaf	Healthy Choice	300
Seafood	Tortilla Crusted Fish	Lean Cuisine	310
Pasta	Tuscan-Style Vegetable Lasagna	Lean Cuisine	310

Pasta	Tortellini w Red Pepper Sauce	Lean Cuisine	310
Pasta	Broccoli Cheddar Rotini	Lean Cuisine	300
Pasta	Three Cheese Ziti Marinara	Smart Ones	300
Pasta	Lasagna Florentine	Smart Ones	300
Seafood	Tortilla Crusted Fish	Lean Cuisine	310
Pasta	Tuscan-Style Vegetable Lasagna	Lean Cuisine	310
Poultry	Chicken Fried Rice	Lean Cuisine	310
Poultry	Orange Chicken	Lean Cuisine	310
Poultry	Chicken Tikka Masala	Lean Cuisine	310
Poultry	Chicken Strips & Fries	Smart Ones	310
Poultry	Chicken Teriyaki	Lean Cuisine	310
Pizza	Thin Crust Pepperoni Pizza	Smart Ones	310
Pasta	Three Cheese Macaroni	Smart Ones	310
Pizza	French Bread Pepperoni Pizza	Lean Cuisine	310
Poultry	Chicken Spinach Mushroom Panini	Lean Cuisine	310
Other	Spicy Beef & Bean Enchilada	Lean Cuisine	310
Poultry	Chicken Fried Rice	Healthy Choice	320
Meat	Sweet & Spicy Korean Beef	Lean Cuisine	320
Pizza	Farmers Market Pizza	Lean Cuisine	320
Pizza	Margherita Pizza	Lean Cuisine	320
Poultry	Chicken Carbonara	Lean Cuisine	330
Poultry	Mango Chicken w Coconut Rice	Lean Cuisine	330
Poultry	Country Fried Chicken	Healthy Choice	330
Other	Cheese & Fire-Roasted Tamale	Lean Cuisine	330
Poultry	Chicken Club Panini	Lean Cuisine	340
Meat	Philly Style Steak & Cheese Panini	Lean Cuisine	350
Poultry	Chicken Parmigiana	Healthy Choice	360
Poultry	Chicken Pecan	Lean Cuisine	370
Poultry	Sweet & Sour Chicken	Healthy Choice	390
Pizza	Supreme Pizza	Lean Cuisine	390

Appendix C
Frozen Food Safety

Increasingly, food giants like ConAgra, Nestlé and others that supply Americans with processed foods concede that they cannot ensure the safety of their food products. Frozen foods pose a particularly serious safety problem because unsuspecting consumers buy frozen foods for their convenience and incorrectly believe that cooking frozen foods is a matter of taste – not safety.

Still the food industry says that extensive outbreaks of food-borne illness are rare, even though it is well-known that most of the millions of cases of food-borne illness every year go unreported or are not traced to the source. For example, each year approximately 40,000 cases of salmonella poisoning are reported in the United States – but perhaps as many as one million cases go unreported. How could this happen? First, the supply chain for ingredients in processed foods – from flour to fruits and vegetables to flavorings – is becoming more complex and global in the drive to keep food costs down. As a result, government and industry officials concede that almost every food ingredient is now a potential carrier of pathogens. A further complication is that a large number of food companies subcontract processing work to save money and don't require suppliers to test for pathogens. In fact, companies often don't even know who is supplying their ingredients.

In addition, many frozen-food manufacturers have stopped cooking their products at high temperatures, a tactic they call the "kill step," which is intended to eliminate any lingering microbes. Frequently this process step turns some of the frozen food ingredients into mush. So, instead the "kill step" has been shifted to consumers. For example, ConAgra has added food safety instructions to its frozen meals, including the Healthy Choice brand. A typical "frozen-food safety" instruction offers this guidance: "Internal temperature needs to reach 165°F as measured by a food thermometer in several spots."

Moreover, General Mills, now advises consumers to avoid microwaves altogether and cook their frozen pizzas only in a conventional oven. **Bottom line**: To be safe, always cook frozen foods so that the internal temperature reaches 165°F as measured by a good food thermometer.

Appendix D
What You Should Weigh

A convenient way to determine what you should weigh is to use our New BMI-Based Weight vs. Height Chart shown in the following table, where normal weight corresponds to a BMI = 18.6 to 24.9, overweight is for BMI = 25.0 to 29.9 and obese is for BMI = 30.0 to 39.9.

Admittedly the weights in the following table would be difficult for most senior men to achieve. But consider the weights shown to be a goal.

Height	Normal	Overweight	Obese
4' 10"	90 – 119	120 – 142	143 – 191
4' 11"	93 – 123	124 – 148	149 – 197
5' 0"	96 – 127	128 – 152	153 – 204
5' 1"	99 – 131	132 – 158	159 – 211
5' 2"	102 – 135	136 – 163	164 – 218
5' 3"	105 – 140	141 – 169	170 – 225
5' 4"	109 – 144	145 – 173	174 – 232
5' 5"	112 – 149	150 – 180	181 – 239
5' 6"	116 – 154	155 – 185	186 – 247
5' 7"	119 – 159	160 – 191	192 – 254
5' 8"	123 – 163	164 – 196	197 – 262
5' 9"	126 – 168	169 – 202	203–270
5' 10"	130 – 173	174 – 206	207 – 278
5' 11"	134 – 178	179 – 214	215 – 286
6' 0"	137 – 183	184 – 220	221 – 294
6' 1"	141 – 188	189 – 227	228 – 302
6' 2"	145 – 194	195 – 232	233 – 310
6' 3"	149 – 199	200 – 239	240 – 319
6' 4"	152 – 205	206 - 246	247 - 328
6' 5"	157 - 210	211 - 252	253 – 337
6' 6"	161 - 216	217 - 259	260 - 346

Weight loss occurs when your food energy intake is less than the total energy you expend. This difference in calories is referred to as your calorie deficit. How much weight you lose depends on the magnitude of your calorie deficit. Physiologists have long known that to lose one pound requires a deficit of approximately 3,500 Calories. Therefore, if a person's total calorie deficit over time is known, their weight loss over time can be calculated. Fortunately, a more precise determination of the rate of weight loss is possible. Scientists have demonstrated that **weight loss is a function of age, sex, height, weight, physical activity, caloric intake and the duration of the diet (or time on the diet)**. This writer related all these variables in a complex, scientifically based, energy-weight-control equation, published in the *American Journal of Clinical Nutrition,*, and subsequently published a set of 60 Weight Loss Prediction tables in the paperback *The Computer Diet* (now published by NoPaperPress). In this book you will find an abridged set of six Weight Loss Prediction tables specifically for senior men.

Selecting the Correct Table

Your first task is to choose the correct Weight Loss Prediction Table. The six Weight Loss Prediction Tables are organized by gender, age and activity level. The three activity levels most applicable to seniors are covered in this text:

1) Sedentary: Inactive most of the day with very little standing or walking.

2) Relatively Inactive: Seated most of the day with about four hours of standing and incidental walking.

3) Moderately Active: To qualify for this category, you have to engage in some form of regular exercise everyday (e.g., taking a brisk three-mile walk).

Use the following table to find the Weight Loss Prediction Table that is applicable to you.

Gender	Age	Activity Level	Table/Page
Men	50 - 65	Sedentary	**E1/147**
	50 - 65	Inactive	**E2/148**
	50 - 65	Active	**E3/149**
	66 - 80	Sedentary	**E4/150**
	66 - 80	Inactive	**E5/151**
	66 - 80	Active	**E6/152**

Weight Loss Prediction Tables

Weight Loss Prediction Example

Consider a 63-year-old man, who is 5' 10" and 200 pounds, is retired but spends most of his free time playing cards and watching TV. How long will it take him to lose 20 pounds?

First he should choose **Table E2 (page 148)** labeled "Weight Loss Prediction for Relatively Inactive Men, Ages 51 - 65 years." Then he would scan the far left of the table and locate his present weight of 200 pounds; from this number he would run a finger horizontally (to the right) until it intersects the vertical column headed by the 20-pound weight loss he desires. The three numbers at the intersection are the time in days to lose 20 pounds, depending on the diet calories he chooses. Specifically, to lose 20 pounds our fictional male's diet calorie options are:

- 1200 Calories per day for 51 days.
- 1500 Calories per day for 63 days.
- 1800 Calories per day for 84 days.

Which alternative should he choose? Health professionals recommend a gradual weight loss of about two pounds per week. In this case, that would mean his diet should last 10 weeks or 70 days, pointing to the 1500-Calorie diet option. Let's assume our fictional dieter decides on 1500 Calories. The above suggests that it will take him about 63 days to lose 20 pounds.

But on the 1200 Calorie diet presented in this book, it will only take our fictional dieter 51 days to lose 20 pounds.

Weight Loss Prediction for Men
(Sedentary - 51 to 65)

Present Weight	Diet Calories	Weight Loss (lbs)							
		10	20	30	40	50	60	70	80
140 lbs	1200	42	89			Numbers in table indicate time in days to lose weight.			
	1500	63	136						
	1800	121	292						
160 lbs	1200	35	74	116					
	1500	49	103	166					
	1800	78	173	294					
180 lbs	1200	31	63	99	137	179	226		
	1500	40	84	133	187	250	323		
	1800	58	125	203	297				
200 lbs	1200	27	56	87	119	155	193	235	
	1500	34	71	101	155	204	259	321	
	1800	47	98	157	223	301			
220 lbs	1200	24	50	77	106	137	169	205	
	1500	30	62	96	133	174	217	266	
	1800	39	82	128	180	238	305		
240 lbs	1200	22	46	70	96	123	151	182	215
	1500	27	55	85	117	152	189	229	273
	1800	34	70	109	152	199	250	308	
260 lbs	1500	20	42	64	87	112	137	164	193
	1800	24	50	77	105	135	167	201	238
	2100	30	62	95	132	171	214	260	312
280 lbs	1500	19	39	59	80	103	126	150	176
	1800	22	45	70	95	122	150	180	213
	2100	27	55	85	117	151	187	226	269

Table E1: Weight Loss, Men, 51 – 65

Weight Loss Prediction for Men
(Relatively Inactive - 51 to 65)

Present Weight	Diet Calories	Weight Loss (lbs)							
		10	20	30	40	50	60	70	80
140 lbs	1200	38	80			Numbers in table indicate time in days to lose weight.			
	1500	54	117						
	1800	93	216						
160 lbs	1200	32	67	105					
	1500	43	91	145					
	1800	64	140	233					
180 lbs	1200	28	58	90	125				
	1500	36	74	117	165				
	1800	49	104	168	244				
200 lbs	1200	25	**51**	79	109	141	176		
	1500	31	**63**	99	138	181	228		
	1800	40	**84**	133	188	252	328		
220 lbs	1200	22	46	70	97	125	154	187	
	1500	27	55	86	119	154	193	236	
	1800	34	71	111	155	204	259	323	
240 lbs	1200	20	42	64	87	112	138	166	196
	1500	24	49	76	105	136	168	204	243
	1800	30	61	95	132	172	216	265	320
260 lbs	1500	19	38	58	80	102	125	151	176
	1800	22	45	69	94	121	150	180	213
	2100	26	54	84	115	149	186	226	
280 lbs	1500	17	35	54	73	94	115	137	161
	1800	20	41	63	86	110	135	162	192
	2100	24	49	75	103	132	164	198	234

Table E2: Weight Loss, Men, 51 – 65

Weight Loss Prediction for Men
(Moderately Active - 51 to 65)

Present Weight	Diet Calories	Weight Loss (lbs)							
		10	20	30	40	50	60	70	80
140 lbs	1200	32	66			Numbers in table indicate time in days to lose weight.			
	1500	42	89						
	1800	62	137						
160 lbs	1200	27	56	87					
	1500	34	71	113					
	1800	45	98	159					
180 lbs	1200	23	48	75	104				
	1500	28	59	93	130				
	1800	36	77	122	174				
200 lbs	1200	21	43	66	91	117	146		
	1500	25	51	79	110	144	181		
	1800	30	63	100	140	186	238		
220 lbs	1200	19	38	59	81	104	129	156	
	1500	22	45	69	96	124	155	189	
	1800	26	54	85	118	154	194	240	
240 lbs	1200	17	35	53	73	94	116	139	164
	1500	20	40	62	85	110	136	164	195
	1800	23	47	74	102	132	165	201	242
260 lbs	1500	16	32	49	67	85	105	126	147
	1800	18	36	56	77	98	121	146	172
	2100	21	42	65	90	116	144	174	207
280 lbs	1500	14	30	45	61	78	96	115	134
	1800	16	33	51	70	89	110	132	155
	2100	19	38	59	81	104	128	154	182

Table E3: Weight Loss, Men, 51 – 65

Weight Loss Prediction for Men
(Sedentary - 66 to 80)

Present Weight	Diet Calories	Weight Loss (lbs)							
		10	20	30	40	50	60	70	80
140 lbs	1200	47	100			Numbers in table indicate time in days to lose weight.			
	1500	74	163						
	1800	173							
160 lbs	1200	39	81	128					
	1500	56	119	193					
	1800	98	222						
180 lbs	1200	33	69	108	151				
	1500	45	95	150	214				
	1800	69	150	248					
200 lbs	1200	29	61	94	130	169	212		
	1500	38	79	124	174	230	293		
	1800	54	114	183	264				
220 lbs	1200	26	54	83	115	148	184	223	
	1500	33	68	106	148	193	242	298	
	1800	44	93	147	207	276	357		
240 lbs	1200	24	49	75	103	132	164	197	233
	1500	29	60	93	129	167	208	253	303
	1800	38	79	123	171	225	286	355	
260 lbs	1500	22	45	69	94	120	148	177	208
	1800	26	54	83	114	146	183	221	262
	2100	33	68	106	147	191	240	294	354
280 lbs	1500	20	41	63	86	110	135	161	189
	1800	24	49	75	103	132	163	196	232
	2100	29	61	94	129	167	207	252	300

Table E4: Weight Loss, Men, 66 – 80

Weight Loss Prediction for Men
(Relatively Inactive - 66 to 80)

Present Weight	Diet Calories	Weight Loss (lbs)							
		10	20	30	40	50	60	70	80
140 lbs	1200	42	89			Numbers in table indicate time in days to lose weight.			
	1500	62	136						
	1800	121	294						
160 lbs	1200	35	73	115					
	1500	48	102	165					
	1800	77	170	291					
180 lbs	1200	30	63	98	136				
	1500	39	83	131	185				
	1800	57	122	198	292				
200 lbs	1200	27	55	85	118	153	191		
	1500	33	70	109	152	200	255		
	1800	45	95	152	217	293			
220 lbs	1200	24	49	76	104	134	167	202	
	1500	29	60	94	130	169	213	261	
	1800	38	79	124	174	231	296		
240 lbs	1200	22	44	68	93	120	148	178	211
	1500	26	54	83	114	147	184	223	266
	1800	33	67	105	146	191	242	298	
260 lbs	1500	20	41	62	85	109	134	161	189
	1800	23	48	74	102	131	162	196	232
	2100	29	59	92	127	194	205	251	301
280 lbs	1500	18	37	57	78	100	122	146	171
	1800	21	44	67	92	118	145	175	206
	2100	26	53	81	112	144	179	217	258

Table E5: Weight Loss, Men, 66 – 80

151

Weight Loss Prediction for Men
(Moderately Active - 66 to 80)

Present Weight	Diet Calories	Weight Loss (lbs)							
		10	20	30	40	50	60	70	80
140 lbs	1200	34	72						
	1500	46	100			Numbers in table			
	1800	72	164			indicate time in			
160 lbs	1200	29	60	94		days to lose weight.			
	1500	37	78	124					
	1800	52	112	184					
180 lbs	1200	25	51	80	111				
	1500	31	64	101	142				
	1800	40	85	137	197				
200 lbs	1200	22	45	70	97	125			
	1500	26	55	86	119	156			
	1800	33	70	110	155	207			
220 lbs	1200	20	40	62	86	111	137	166	
	1500	23	48	74	103	134	167	204	
	1800	28	59	92	129	169	214	266	
240 lbs	1200	18	37	56	77	99	122	147	174
	1500	21	43	66	91	117	146	176	210
	1800	25	51	80	110	143	180	220	265
260 lbs	1500	16	34	52	70	90	111	133	157
	1800	19	39	59	81	105	129	156	184
	2100	22	45	70	97	125	156	189	225
280 lbs	1500	15	31	47	65	83	101	121	142
	1800	17	35	54	74	95	117	140	165
	2100	20	41	63	86	112	137	166	196

Table E6: Weight Loss, Men, 66 – 80

NoPaperPress eBooks and Paperbacks

100-Day Super Diet-1200 Cal*
100-Day Super Diet-1500 Cal*
100-Day No-Cooking Diet-1200 Cal*
100-Day No-Cooking Diet-1500 Cal*
31 Smart Diet-1200 Cal*
90-Day Smart Diet-1500 Cal*
90-Day No-Cooking Diet - 1200 Cal*
90-Day No-Cooking Diet - 1500 Cal*
90-Day Perfect Diet - 1200 Cal*
90-Day Perfect Diet - 1500 Cal*
60-Day Perfect Diet-1200 Cal*
60-Day Perfect Diet-1500 Cal*
50-Day Flex Diet-1200 Cal*
50-Day Flex Diet-1500 Cal*
30-Day Quick Diet - Women*
30-Day Quick Diet for Men*
30-Day No-Cooking Diet*
30-Day Diet for Women - Metric*
30-Day Diet for Men - Metric*
25 Day Easy Diet-1200 Cal*
25 Day Easy Diet-1500 Cal*
25-Day No-Cooking Diet
10-Day Express Diet
10-Day No-Cooking Diet*
7-Day Diet for Women*
7-Day Diet for Men*
7-Day No-Cooking Diets*
90-Day Gluten-Free Diet-1200 Cal*
90-Day Gluten-Free Diet-1500 Cal*
30-Day Gluten-Free Quick Diet*
30-Day Gluten-Free No-Cooking*
7-Day Diet for Women - Metric*
7-Day Diet for Men - Metric
7-Day Gluten-Free Express Diet*
7-Day Gluten-Free No-Cooking Diet*
90-Day Vegetarian Diet-1200 Cal*
90-Day Vegetarian Diet-1500 Cal*
30-Day Vegetarian Diet*
7-Day Vegetarian Diet*
Weight Loss for Women*
Weight Loss for Women - Metric
Weight Loss for Women - UK
Weight Loss for Men*
Maximum Weight Loss - 1200 Cal*
Maximum Weight Loss - 1500 Cal*

Weight Loss for Men - Metric*
Maximum Weight Loss- 1200 Cal*
Maximum Weight Loss- 1500 Cal*
Weight Control - U.S. Edition*
Weight Control - Metric. Edition
Prof Weight Control Women - U.S.
Prof Weight Control Women - Metric
Prof Weight Control Men - U.S.
Prof Weight Control Men - Metric
Weight Maintenance - U.S. Ed*
Weight Maintenance - Metric. Ed*
Weight Maintenance - UK Ed
Weight Loss for Senior Men*
Weight Loss for Senior Women*
Eat Smart - U.S. Edition*
Eat Smart - Metric Edition
30-Day Mediterranean Diet
Exercise Smart - U.S. Edition*
Exercise Smart - Metric Edition
Exercise Smart - UK Edition*
Total Fitness - U.S. Edition
Total Fitness - Metric Edition
Total Fitness - UK Edition
Total Fitness for Women-U.S. Ed*
Total Fitness for Women - Metric
Total Fitness for Women - UK Ed
Total Fitness for Men - U.S. Ed*
Total Fitness for Men- Metric Ed*
Total Fitness for Men - UK Ed
Senior Fitness - U.S. Edition*
Senior Fitness - Metric Edition*
Senior Fitness - UK Edition*
Computer Diet - U.S. Edition*
Computer Diet - Metric Ed*
Reliable Weight Loss - U.S. Ed
101 Weight Loss Tips*
101 Healthy Eating Tips*
101 Lifelong Fitness Tips*
101 Weight Maintenance Tips
101 Weight Loss Recipes
101 GF Weight Loss Recipes
101 Veggie Weight Loss Recipes*
30-Day Mediterranean Diet*
90-Day Mediterranean Diet - 1200 Cal*
90-Day Mediterranean Diet - 1500 Cal*

* These titles are available as both ebooks and paperbacks. Our ebooks are sold by Amazon, Apple, Google, Barnes & Noble and Kobo, but our paperbacks are only sold by Amazon.

Disclaimer

This book offers general meal planning, nutrition and weight control information. It is not a medical manual and the author does not claim to be medically qualified. The material in this book is not intended to be a substitute for medical counseling. Everyone should have a medical checkup before beginning a weight loss program. Moreover, the physician conducting the medical exam should be made aware of and should approve the specific weight control program planned. Additionally, while the author and publisher have made every effort to ensure the accuracy of the information in this book, they make no representations or warranties regarding its accuracy or completeness. Further, neither the author nor publisher assume liability for any medical problems that might result from applying the methods in this book, or for any loss of profit, or any other commercial damages, including but not limited to special, incidental, consequential or other damages, and any such liability is hereby expressly disclaimed.